The Autoimmune Protocol Diet Instant Pot Cookbook

The Most Healing Instant Pot Recipes to Beat Autoimmune Diseases

Written by Bobby Stone

TABLE OF CONTENTS

INTRODUCTION

There are many different motives for wanting to change your diet. If you're like me, I bet you never grew up eating all the healthy foods we should have been hard-wired to eat from childhood. Perhaps you're looking to lose weight, but if you're looking to start the AIP/Paleo diet then it's likely your biggest reason is your health. There are a number of reasons why the average American diet is bad for someone with an autoimmune disease, but the number one reason has to do with inflammation. Because most autoimmune diseases are caused by inflammation, consuming additional inflammatory substances isn't the best idea. Sadly, the majority of the American diet—white sugar, white bread, refined/processed foods, artificial ingredients, GMOs, etc. - is highly inflammatory.

You're in the right place if you want to address your autoimmune disease naturally. Right now, a life without symptoms or prescriptions may seem impossible to you. I'm passionate about helping others heal from autoimmune diseases because I've experienced the frustration and suffering they cause. However, my mom got her life back after years with a debilitating autoimmune disease called Ulcerative Colitis. Now, she's medication-free with no signs of the disease, thanks to a friend who suggested the nutritional autoimmune protocol.

If you've been diagnosed with an autoimmune disease, I want to reach out to you through this book, hold your hands, and tell you with all the conviction in my heart, "Please start the autoimmune protocol. I know it seems overwhelming. Maybe your symptoms don't seem bad enough to change your lifestyle. But your symptoms are the voice of your wise body, asking you to make drastic changes." It's helped my mom and it can most definitely help you if you persistently follow this diet. The Autoimmune Protocol diet, often referred to as the AIP or Paleo diet, is a healing diet that works as one component of a successful treatment plan in helping most people suffering from an autoimmune disease find a path to recovery.

Chapter 1:
The AIP Diet

What is Autoimmune Protocol (AIP)?

The Autoimmune Protocol was originally developed by Dr. Loren Cordain and Robb Wolf (see the "*Autoimmune Caveat*" in The Paleo Solution) as a variation of the Paleo diet, to help those with autoimmune diseases.

The idea is to eliminate foods that can "irritate and damage the intestines of people", even though these eliminated foods are typically allowed on a Paleo diet.

Remember that AIP is an eliminate-and-then-reintroduce diet! So, the idea is to eliminate all foods on the "not allowed" list for at least 30-60 days (30 days is generally suggested by most people, but some people do 60 days to make sure – Robb states "a month or two" in his book), and then to re-introduce one food at a time to see how your body reacts.

The idea behind the eliminate-and-then-reintroduce approach is that your body reacts badly with most (but not all) of the "not allowed" foods. However, you won't be able to tell which ones you react badly to unless you first eliminate all of them, very strictly, for the 30-60 day period.

The goal of the AIP diet is to remove foods that could trigger inflammation or harm gut health, and instead eat nutrient-dense foods that promote health; such as bone broth, liver, fermented foods, high-quality meats, and leafy and cruciferous vegetables.

Based on a general Paleo template, the AIP diet focuses on removing foods such as grains, legumes, dairy, industrial seed oils, refined sugar, eggs, nightshades (like eggplants, tomatoes, and potatoes), coffee, alcohol, nuts, and seeds.

The AIP diet routinely gets a lot of attention, even in the mainstream media. Some question if the diet is a legitimate way to manage an autoimmune disease, asserting that "a lot of it doesn't make much biological sense."

How does AIP differ from Paleo?

For the most part, the 30-60 day elimination component of AIP is a stricter version of Paleo. So, you do a pure Paleo diet, and then just eliminate the additional "not allowed" foods for AIP. After the 30-60 day period, you should slowly and considerately reintroduce the "not allowed" foods back into your Paleo diet.

After you've tried to reintroduce all the "not allowed" foods back into your Paleo diet, you will keep doing the Paleo diet and keep eliminating any of the foods that caused you problems when you tried to reintroduce them. For example, if your autoimmune condition worsened when you reintroduced eggs back into your diet after the 30-60 day elimination period, then you would need to keep eggs out of your Paleo diet - even though most people on a Paleo diet eat lots of eggs!

Benefits of AIP Diet

Anyone who has battled with autoimmune disease knows it's not something you can heal with a pill or a procedure. When my mom was dealing with autoimmune disease she often described it as feeling like she was living in an alternate reality— like any disorienting experience, it can come with its fair share of uncertainty, anxiety, and fear. But when we moved past the suffering and denial, which often comes before embracing the diagnosis of an autoimmune disease, we were able to become more receptive to healing in alternative ways.

While simply following the Autoimmune Protocol diet is a starting point to beat autoimmune diseases, I have seen it trigger a paradigm shift as it helps you eliminate poor decisions too. It forces you to change your everyday habits and say "yes" to the things that will help you heal and "no, thank you" to that which harms. Overtime, I watched the way my mom's thought process transform—I noticed how she shopped differently, the wise choice of foods she went for, consciously choosing the alternatives for the foods she loved, drinking smoothies she hated, how much more active she became. I could only imagine when she went to bed that she was battling through the lens of, "Is this helping me to heal?" and mustering the will to adjust her mindset accordingly.

It takes significant discipline to heal in this way. It's so inspiring for me to watch my mom go from feeling hopeless, awful, hurt, and defeated to a place of empowerment as she learned to embrace and respond to the disease rather than neglect and feed it. The transformation of this spirit can feel damn close to miraculous to watch! It's such a gift for me to be able to support others just like my mom on this journey, and reflect her victory to them. Here are some of the things I regularly saw my mom developing as we embarked on her healing journeys — many of which are not even directly related to diet.

AUTHENTICITY

Adopting the autoimmune protocol as part of our identity is by far one of the most challenging parts of AIP. It takes grit, persistence, determination, and discipline to eventually say to yourself, "this is who I am and this is the new, healthier me,", even if it's just turning down a piece of cake or a beer at a friend's birthday party. Our cultural norm is to do what is comfortable, and that's a very powerful system to buck. I love seeing people embrace what's truly meant for them and own it.

A SENSE OF WHAT MATTERS MOST

Over time, people dealing with autoimmune disease inevitably learn that they can't have or do it all—for the body to heal itself, something has to give. I have worked in the hospice world for over 4 years and I've seen different perspectives of life from the vantage point of the deathbed. I've often asked clients to list at least 20 things that were most important in their lives, and why these things were so important. I did this because I have always believed that when you have a strong desire for something, you will do everything within your power to see it through. I hoped to invoke that fighting spirit for patients to see them reverse their disease through a positive mental attitude. The same goes when applying the AIP diet. Sooner or later, your relationship, job, habit, or food that is causing stress on the immune system has got to fade because of your mental attitude of what's most important.

GRIT

Embracing the Autoimmune Protocol can be hard work! Skipping out on freshly baked bread, not eating Aunt Susie's famous stuffing at Thanksgiving, rejecting that fresh summer cocktail...when you are constantly faced with the challenges of honoring what your body needs, it takes a gritty effort to stay on track. The line "thanks, but no thanks," becomes your predominant attitude. The Autoimmune Protocol doesn't promise a quick fix — it's not a 30-day diet. It doesn't save time and it's not convenient, especially when you're starting out. But it's sure as hell worth it. It's the opposite of everything we're sold in the diet industry! Anyone who has stuck through an elimination/reintroduction process knows that removing all foods that may be exacerbating your problems is difficult and can take time. Ultimately, it depends on you. Your faith, attitude, and persistence, and knowledge that if you slip up it takes perseverance to pick yourself up and keep going. Silence any discouraging thoughts and protect your mind as well as your body. Even being diagnosed in the first place can feel like a laborious process, often involving worry and doubts from family and friends. Eating and living this way is a choice of lifestyle because we are determined to heal in direct and indirect ways, which will make loved ones feel inspired by such transformation. Developing the grit to stick with it and materialize the benefits is one of the most powerful and affirming shift I saw in my mom's journey to recovery.

SELF-AWARENESS

It is more challenging to become successful with the Autoimmune Protocol without frequently checking in on yourself. It is essential to assess, analyze, test, and note the things that work and those that don't work. Take the time to figure out what works and doesn't work for your body. We are often told in our culture to just do whatever feels good, whatever we're told, or whatever everyone else is doing. But with the AIP, you cannot rely on any external claims or guidance. You have to be your own guide as you check labels on food, personal care products, and cleaning products to figure out what works for you. It's like trying to put together a very complicated puzzle that is unique to each person. A strong self-awareness and a positive mental attitude are essential components to succeed with the AIP.

EMPOWERMENT

As you develop new awareness and the ability to care for yourself, you start to take your health into your own hands. I've seen it first-hand watching my mom experience the victim role — focusing on the unfairness of her diagnosis and wondering if she had what it takes to heal — she flipped this to embrace the power and knowledge to make herself feel better. I remember my uncle giving her his usual pep talk and mentioning how no-one was responsible for her health but her; and how only she, not a doctor, could make herself healthy again. Since then, it was like a light bulb was switched on. Suddenly her attitude became a means for healing.

GROWTH MINDSET

Once people start to unlock some success in their journey with autoimmune disease and begin honing in on what works for them and what doesn't, there is a temptation to assume they have it all solved. But anyone who has been dealing with an autoimmune disease long enough will tell you that the pursuit of wellness needs continuous adjustment. Learning how to trust in one's body and embrace the idea that things may not always be perfect is difficult, but a growth mindset prepares you for new changes.

CONTENTMENT

While the AIP is largely focused on diet, we all know that health and wellness benefits don't only come from food. When you continue down this path, you'll recognize that there is a history of health abuse in the form of chronic stress, caloric restriction, soul-draining jobs, negative self-talk, or excessive exercise. As well as looking at your diet, we recommend you focus on stress management, improving relationships, joining meditation or yoga classes, jotting down 10 things a day that you're grateful for, using strategies to set better boundaries at work, and taking time to exercise on a routine basis — these practices will have a dramatic impact on your happiness. Getting a handle on the disease and finding more happiness in your life will continue to move you through a giant leap of the healing process because you'll feel less stressed, and we, ourselves are much better at healing our own bodies than anyone or anything else.

SELF-RESPECT

Self-respect is crucial in the healing process; it's putting your needs before the wants of other people and yourself. Folks who struggle with self-respect come across as very indifferent and look externally for reasons to make changes; wanting others to take on their burdens, making excuses as to why they can't, and killing the truth that they can, etc. This usually leads to a tug of war effect, where sometimes they do absolutely wonderfully and eat well, but at other times they lose faith and let their mental struggles push them backwards. This is natural, but the truth is that the path to a more significant change over time can't come from a place of self-aggression. It comes from self-perseverance. When my mom lost her faith I reminded her of how she used to look when she was younger and she stuck photos around the house to remind her of who she actually was and would be again – healthy, strong and beautiful. It's such a joy to see my mom make this shift over time.

Like any struggle in life, autoimmune disease gives us an opportunity to shift our values. It gives us a purpose. We get to learn new skills, experiences, and knowledge, which all give us new ways of showing up in the world. I had a patient say to me recently, "I wish that I could just erase all the hard stuff I've dealt with and not remember it." While I agreed that it would be nice to not have gone through pain in the past, I tried to shine a light on the transformation she'd experienced by dealing with hardship and noticing the benefits that others haven't been blessed to see. I believe that we make our true mark on this world when things aren't perfectly easy — and that means embracing our struggles. I'd love to hear about your reflections on your autoimmune journey. How have you seen shifts in your values or character? Let's celebrate those wins! Cheers to resiliency!

Chapter 2: Basics of the AIP Diet

Does AIP work?

I can personally say that this diet has worked wonders for my mom. It has helped to distinguish the triggering so-called foods that my mom "loved" and now she is pretty used to new alternatives. Ultimately, I put her transformation down to her sheer will and attitude as there were more complimentary things she adopted to her lifestyle. Despite my experience, there are minimal scientific studies proving the efficacy of AIP; primarily because the concept is relatively new and there's not a lot of funding for this kind of research. On the other hand, anecdotal evidence suggests that it works quite well. In fact, Sarah Ballantyne states that AIP "is appropriate for everyone with diagnosed autoimmune disorders or with suspected autoimmune diseases." It's certainly a long-term solution worth giving a shot.

Who Should Try AIP?

Based on evidence of the number of people who've spoken about their autoimmune conditions, I think most people find just sticking to a very pure Paleo diet helps with their conditions. In particular, I've heard from a lot of people who have improved their Rheumatoid Arthritis with just a Paleo diet (without attempting AIP).

However, even for those people, a Paleo autoimmune protocol may improve their autoimmune condition even more (read Eileen's story comparing how much better her Rheumatoid Arthritis got on AIP rather than on the GAPS diet, and Tara's story on how she had to modify her Paleo diet to improve her Hidradenitis Suppurativa).

And for those people (like my mom) whose autoimmune conditions don't improve with Paleo, trying AIP is definitely an option to consider! The main downside to AIP is that it is very restrictive, and you have to be very strict during the entire period or you'll risk going to all that trouble for nothing.

So, if you're considering doing AIP, make sure to give yourself at least 60 days to test it out - 30 days elimination followed by a 30 day reintroduction period. Because the diet is so restrictive, it's best you don't eat takeouts during that period. This has been one of my mom's biggest deterrents to trying AIP so far. Also, be prepared to face the fact that AIP is TOUGH! I've always recognized that AIP is tough. I personally have a hard time imagining life without most of the spices that I cook with. To that end, reading Eileen's and Melissa's accounts have made it all the more real for me.

The ABCs of AIP: A Beginners Guide To The Autoimmune Protocol

The AIP diet works by removing inflammatory foods from your diet and replacing them with a higher consumption of nutrient-dense, gut healing, immune-boosting foods. Starting AIP can be daunting, especially because most of the foods cut out with AIP are staples in the typical American diet. But as someone who first-hand knows how you can use the AIP diet to recover from an autoimmune disease, I can tell you that every day of missing bread is worth it.

AIP means no gluten, no grains, no legumes (beans), no dairy, no sugar, no nightshades (things like white potatoes, eggplant, peppers, and tomatoes that irritate your gut), and no alcohol—this is also the basic Paleo principle.

A = Always Listen to Your Body

According to the AIP guidelines you should be able to handle all forms of natural or organic meats, but my digestive tract doesn't sit well with certain kinds of beef. You must understand that just because this is a healing diet, doesn't mean it's universal. If you drink coconut milk and don't feel great, or are struggling to consume the number of calories you need without grains, then think outside the box. There are a lot of substitutes for milk you can try out: flax, almond, cashew, hazelnut, etc (just steer clear of soy for now), and the market for grain-free and gluten-free products is vastly growing. Just make sure that you check the list of ingredients before you buy something marketed as grain-free, gluten-free, or dairy-free because it might not be good for you.

And if you're hungry, eat! Don't be afraid to look up some recipes for AIP snacks, or have a piece of fruit or some homemade sweet potato fries.

B = Books, Blogs, and Bone Broth

With the development of technology,there are tons of cookbooks, online communities, and food blogs dedicated to AIP and Paleo diets and lifestyles, so you're never alone when you're searching for something to eat. It's never been easier to learn new tips and tricks for navigating this new phase of your life. All it takes is a little googling or a quick trip to Amazon to find tons of resources for helping to be AIP. There's plenty of AIP blogs, dessert AIP blogs, mom AIP blogs, athlete AIP blogs, the list goes on and on!

Don't shy away from the weird. Bone broth might sound like something cannibalistic witches drink, but it's another name for a basic soup stock made with the bones of animals. Think of it this way; if you ever make home-made soup with a whole chicken or any other bone-in meat, you've made a version of bone broth. Bone broth is amazing for healing your gut and is filled with wonderful nutrients and proteins to ensure that you have a well-rounded diet. Also, it's just freaking delicious!

C = Cooking is Your New Best Friend

AIP meals at restaurants can be hard to come by, which means if you're eating out you'll be eating a lot of salads and some of them will be sad, it's just a fact of life—don't get me wrong, you'll also find some amazing salads, but sad salads are just a reality that us Paleo and AIP people face. Because it can be difficult to eat out, cooking your meals will take on whole new importance in your life. By no means does this mean you need to go out and become a five-star chef - AIP cooking can be really easy! Here are just a few easy AIP recipes to get you started and excited.

Chapter 3: Starting the AIP Diet

Understanding a leaky gut

A discussion of a leaky gut is required to understand the autoimmune protocol. You need to know how food is impacting your body, and whether it's perpetuating or healing the disease — this will keep you alert and motivated enough to make drastic, sustained lifestyle changes.

Here is a leaky gut described in a nutshell:

The small intestine, where nutrients are absorbed, is supposed to have tight cell junctions to separate the chyme (food turns into chyme in the stomach) from the bloodstream. But a chain of factors, including stress and environmental toxins, are causing the tight junctions to degrade.

Once the connections between intestinal cells have become weakend, the undigested proteins and bacterial toxins escapes into the bloodstream. This leads to a heightened state of inflammation, allergies, and eventually autoimmunity.

Autoimmune symptoms dissipate when the gut heals. Inflammative toxins and proteins no longer end up in the bloodstream, and the body neutralizes its own attack on the tissue.

Bulk cooking prevents breakdowns on Autoimmune Paleo

Food prepping and cooking in large batches is one of the most important tips for the autoimmune paleo protocol. It helps to prepare and plan ahead before stressing about what to eat and piling more workload on than neccessary. I personally set aside an hour or two, twice a week, to crank out meals for the rest of the week. Here's what one of my cooking sessions might look like:

I'll make meatballs with 3 lbs of ground beef, freeze half the batch after cool down. This gives me about 6 portions worth of protein in the fridge for a couple days and 6 more in the freezer.

I prepare around 3 butternut squashes which I roast to make butternut squash puree and then freeze half the batch.

I'll freeze 2 bunches of ripe bananas for smoothies.

And I'll also start a fresh batch of bone broth.

I may also make a double batch of my Grain-Free Gravy recipe and freeze half. This is a perfect all-purpose autoimmune paleo sauce.

Meal planning is key for Autoimmune Paleo

Although meal planning sounds time-intensive and complicated, this simple task takes only a few minutes out of your day and saves you from mealtime distress. When I plan meals, I start by planning one dinner at a time. I prepare just enough for that dinner so that I have at least three meals pre-planned. This way, we can have some easy breakfasts and lunches. I also plan some easy "reheat meals." For example, I'll make a big pot of soup that I can quickly reheat at mealtimes.

Basic meal planning entails writing down a grocery list, making notes about when you need to thaw out meat or frozen foods, and how much of something you will cook. You will also want to briefly outline a main dish and side dish for each meal or simply designate a meal as "leftovers." Remember - cook in bulk so that you have leftovers!

Find additional Autoimmune Paleo Recipes on Pinterest

When it comes to the Autoimmune Paleo protocol, Pinterest offers a one-stop-shop to easily find hundreds of AIP-friendly recipes. You can go to the search bar and type in "autoimmune paleo", then narrow your search by pins or boards.

Set a date to start the Autoimmune Paleo Protocol

The Autoimmune Paleo Protocol provides powerful healing potential, but it is not a flexible routine. As scary as it may sound, there is no room for cheating during this temporary healing period. It's all about giving the intestinal lining an uninterrupted chance for healing, and incorporating an inflammatory food binge-eating session can flare up the disease or drag the healing progress backward.

If you are currently experiencing symptoms of autoimmune diseases, I recommend starting Autoimmune Protocol as soon as possible. The longer autoimmunity goes unaddressed, the more damage it creates and the more time you will need to heal. If your disease is less aggressive, you have more flexibility with starting the protocol. You may choose to wait a month or two until things are quieter at work so you have more energy to devote to the protocol.

Forget the concept of "breakfast food"

One common pitfall of the Autoimmune Paleo Protocol is attempting to find suitable breakfast foods. The simplest solution? Forget the concept of what breakfast SHOULD be. Who says that cereal, pancakes or granola bars are a mandatory way to start the morning; or worse, a healthy way?

Stay centered: don't take flack!

Many of you may be in the same boat I was when I started a grain-free healing diet to address my autoimmune prevention. Fortunately, my immediate family was very supportive because it was something I'd experienced first hand with my mom, but things were challenging with friends coming out with rather thoughtless remarks. Things like: "Why can't you go out to eat with us? Just one meal at a restaurant isn't going to kill you." Or "Seriously, you can't eat this either?" Or "I can't believe you use lard when cooking. That stuff is so bad for you."

Don't forget the Autoimmune Paleo lifestyle changes

"How do I live a normal life and follow the Autoimmune Paleo Protocol?" If your "normal life" is munching a morning granola bar in the car and grabbing a pizza with coworkers after work, then the short answer is "You don't."

Autoimmune Paleo is a lifestyle change, but it will change your life. On this healing journey, you will discover strength you didn't know you had. You will discover gifts which you will use to support others in their own healing.

There are some tradeoffs, but it's worth it. You'll outgrow your old, normal life.

Although changes may seem jolting at first, I promise things will smooth out into routine quickly. Here are some of the lifestyle changes you may need to introduce:

Packing your lunch for work (no more fast food or takeout leftovers)

Prioritizing sleep

Regular grocery trips to keep the fridge stocked with fresh produce

Getting a daily dose of sunlight for vitamin D

Finding stress management routines that work for you

Know how to re-introduce foods

What do you get when you combine a "Recovering Perfectionist" with the GAPS Diet or Autoimmune Paleo Protocol or other forms of an elimination diet?

You get someone who is great at removing foods from their diet, and following the food rules, but who is hesitant to add foods back into their diet.

Chapter 4: Choosing the Right Food for You

How to Choose the Right Food and Avoid the Wrong Ones

Each autoimmune disease are different from one another. Yet scientific research suggests the power of plants is useful to help alleviate common symptoms and to ultimately heal the body. At first, the AIP diet can be overwhelming and challenging. Luckily, our purpose serves to eliminate any ignorance on the subject matter, create an easy guideline, and make you aware of what IS possible. It is imperretive you follow these tips to ensure your success.

Start with basic paleo principles

Set a disciplined target to eliminate gluten, grains, legumes, dairy, sugar, and alcohol for the first 30-60 days.

Gluten is inflammatory for the gut and should be removed from the diet for anyone with autoimmune disorders.

Grains and legumes should be removed to avoid anti-nutrients like phytic acid and inflammatory lectins.

Sugar and alcohol are removed because they are highly inflammatory and do not bring any nutritional value or healing properties to the table.

Nightshade vegetables such as peppers, eggplants, and tomatoes should be avoided completely. These are highly inflammative and trigger joint pain, skin irritation, and gut discomfort.

Avoid eggs

Eggs are eliminated because the proteins and enzymes in eggs (the whites in particular) can work their way through the gut lining during the digestion process. Although this can occur in healthy people as well, those with autoimmune conditions are more receptive to the negative effects. The egg particulate matter finds its way through the barrier of the gut lining easily and infiltrates the bloodstream, stimulating the immune system and causing reactivity.

Avoid all nuts and seeds

Nuts and seeds are high in lectins, phytates, and other anti-nutrients that you must avoid. They are one of the most allergenic types of foods and can cause sensitivities in people struggling with autoimmunity. Moreover, the ratio of omega-3 to omega-6 fatty acids is suboptimal in most nuts and seeds. Nuts contain a high amount of omega-6 fatty acids which are pro-inflammatory and likely to do more harm to your body.

Keep fruit to a minimum

Try to consume fruits - between one or two servings per day. This will keep the blood sugar level stable and also help you avoid taking in too much fructose, which can be irritating for the gut.

Avoid food additives like guar gum and carrageenan

These additives bring no health benefits and contribute to leaky gut. Other additives they contain, such as nitrites, are inflammative for the body and can also be allergenic.

Avoid non-steroidal anti-inflammatory medications

Avoiding NSAIDs is about attempting to heal the gut lining, as this is critical in managing autoimmune disorders. Avoiding these can be tricky because many medical suggestions for autoimmune disorders, such as rheumatoid arthritis, chronic pain syndromes, and acute bouts of thyroiditis, are to use these. Before removing any medications from your regimen, be sure to discuss matters with your medical provider.

How Long Should I Follow The AIP Diet?

One of the most crucial components to fulfilling AIP success for your health is to set a time period and track your symptoms over a number of weeks within that period (You can use a journal, calendar, or notebook). How long you choose to stay on the AIP is 100% up to you and should depend on how you feel following the diet.

A strict elimination period of at least 30-60 days is recommended, but many people stay on the protocol for months until they start seeing the resolution of their autoimmune symptoms.

By setting a timeline for your elimination diet, you can focus on the healing aspects of the diet and stay motivated with an endpoint in sight.

The 4R Approach

The simple '4R approach' is like four commandments to avoiding and improving autoimmune-related diseases.

Remove all toxins and gut irritants like alcohol, caffeine, drugs (over the counter, antibiotics, etc.), gluten, dairy, corn, soy, legumes, industrial seed oils, and sugar.

Replace them with healthy and healing foods like those found on the paleo diet, superfoods like bone broth, and fermented foods.

Repair with specific supplements such as L-glutamine, zinc, omega-3s, and vitamins A, C, D, and E.

Restore with healthy bacteria and probiotics (25-100 billion units), digestive enzymes, hydrochloric acid, and soluble fiber.

How To Re-introduce Foods

While the AIP diet may help you find out which foods you react to, the strict autoimmune protocol is not necessarily meant to be followed for life.

After removing some, or better yet, all of these restricted foods for three to four weeks, then you can start to reintroduce them very slowly one at a time.

On the first day of reintroduction, you may decide to include a dairy product, such as cheese. After this first day of reintroduction, you'll want to wait two to three days before reintroducing another food. This is because it can often take 24-72 hours for your body to have a response to what you've eaten.

Despite some of the more obvious physical reactions, monitor and pay attention to your mood, energy, sleeping habits, digestion, headaches and sinuses, bloating, and cognitive function.

It's highly recommended you use a journal throughout this process to record your results, measure progress, and to refer to later on.

Chapter 5: Breakfast Recipes

AIP Friendly Breakfast Porridge {Instant Pot Option}

Servings: 1-2

Prep Time: 5 mins

Cook Time: 15 mins

Total Time: 20 mins

Ingredients

- 2–3 tbsp lightly toasted sunflower seeds or 1 tbsp tahini (For seed substitute, use an additional 2 tbsp of coconut flakes or coconut butter [grounded])
- 2 tbsp unsweetened shredded coconut
- 1 tbsp chia seed or flaxseed (omit for AIP or substitute with 1 tbsp collagen/ gelatin powder)
- 1/2 tsp cinnamon
- 1 tsp ginger, ground
- Pinch of turmeric, ground
- Pinch of sea salt
- 1/2 cup water or coconut milk, more if needed
- 1 cup squash, cooked (ex: butternut squash or kabocha/ or acorn squash).
- If using Instant Pot you will need additional coconut oil or ghee and water
- Optional hemp protein or collagen
- Pure maple syrup or raw honey

Extra toppings:

- Tart cherries (pitted), blueberries, pomegranate seeds, sesame seed, and/or coconut cream or yogurt to top.

Instructions

1. Peel and chop your squash into large pieces.
2. Place in the instant pot with 1 tbsp or less of coconut oil.
3. Add in a pinch of cinnamon and nutmeg and sauté for 5 minutes, turning the squash.
4. Once the squash is coated, Add 1/3 cup of water to Pressure Cooker cooking pot and lock on lid and close pressure valve.
5. Cook on Manual high pressure for 5-6 minutes.
6. Allow a 10-minute natural pressure release. Or use a quick release if short on time. Release the lid, drain the water then puree the squash with a hand blender.
7. Mix in your other ingredients (dry mix and tahini/sesame mix) and a splash of milk (no dairy). Stir all together. Place the lid back on and keep it on warm mode until ready to serve. See notes for meal prep.

Nutrition

- Calories: 331
- Fat 17.7g
- Carbohydrate 43.1g
- Protein 7g

Autoimmune-Friendly Apple Pie Applesauce

Servings: 6

Prep Time: 10 mins

Cook Time: 20 mins

Total Time: 30 mins

Ingredients

- 3 1/2 lb assorted sweet and tart apples (such as Gala, Granny Smith, and Fuji)
- 2 tsp lemon juice freshly squeezed
- 2 tsp ghee
- 1/4 tsp ground cinnamon (per serving)
- 1/8 tsp ground allspice
- 1/8 tsp fine sea salt

Instructions

1. Peel, core, and slice the apples. Place the apples, 3/4 cup water, and the lemon juice, ghee, cinnamon, allspice, and salt in an electric pressure cooker.
2. If using an Instant Pot, secure the lid and turn the valve to pressure.
3. Select the Manual or Pressure Cook button and set it to high pressure for 5 minutes.
4. Once the timer has sounded, let the machine release the pressure on its own; it will take about 15 minutes. (Alternatively, carefully release the pressure manually.) Remove the lid.
5. Using an immersion blender or conventional blender, pulse the applesauce to your desired consistency. Serve warm with cinnamon sprinkled on top, or refrigerate and enjoy chilled.
6. Store the applesauce in an airtight container in the refrigerator for 10 days or in an airtight container in the freezer for 6 months.
7. Allow it to thaw overnight in the refrigerator before serving.
8. If desired, reheat in a saucepan over medium-low heat for 8 to 10 minutes, until heated through.

Nutrition

- Calories: 243
- Fat: 10g
- Carbohydrate: 36.8g
- Protein: 4.6g

Perfect Baked Sweet Potatoes in the Pressure Cooker and Oven

Servings: 1

Prep Time: 1 min

Cook Time: 45 mins

Total Time: 46 mins

Ingredients

- 1 sweet potato per serving
- 1 cup boiling water

Instructions

1. Wash the sweet potatoes well. Poke each with a fork a few times.
2. Pour 1 cup of hot water in your pressure cooker.
3. Place a steaming rack or basket in the pot.
4. Make sure the water is beneath the level of the rack.
5. Place the potatoes on the rack, out of the water.
6. How much time you pressure cook them will depend on the size of the sweet potatoes.
7. Lock your lid in place and bring to high pressure.
8. It doesn't matter how many potatoes you are cooking; set the timer according to the size of the largest potato.
9. Cook at high pressure for the time listed for your size of sweet potatoes.
10. Then remove from heat or turn your electric PC off.
11. Allow the pressure to come down naturally for 10 minutes.
12. Quick-release the pressure if necessary after 10 minutes.
13. Check the potatoes by poking down to the center with a fork.
14. If they seem hard in the middle, return them to the cooker, and pressure cook them for another minute or two.
15. Quick-release the pressure and check again. They should be done, but repeat if necessary.
16. While the pressure is coming down, preheat your oven to 400F.
17. Place the sweet potatoes on a baking sheet and bake for 10-15 minutes.
18. Serve warm.

Nutrition

- Calories
- Fat 0.3g
- Carbohydrates 37.3g
- Protein 3.6g

Easy Instant Pot Apple Butter (w/Gluten-Free Toast)

Servings: 1 cup

Prep Time: 5 mins

Cook Time: 2 hrs

Cooling Time: 3 hrs (Can store 2 weeks in fridge/3 months in freezer)

Total Time: 5 hrs 5 mins

Ingredients

- 1/4 cup water
- 1/2 cup honey
- 6 apples roughly chopped (pears are a great substitute!)
- 1/2 teaspoon ground cinnamon
- 1/8 teaspoon ground cloves

Instructions

1. Add all the ingredients into the Instant Pot.
2. Stir to combine and then cover.
3. Pressure cook for 10 minutes.
4. Let sit for about 10 minutes and then allow to vent (quick release).
5. Make sure that the red stopper has dropped before you remove the cover.
6. Next set the instant pot to Sauté on low.
7. Allow to sauté for 1 hour 30 minutes or so while stirring occasionally.
8. Use the immersion blender to puree the apples.
9. If you don't have an immersion blender, you can use a regular blender or food processor.
10. Either way, you'll need to take the apple mixture out of the instant pot to puree.
11. Remember, the mixture will firm up slightly once it's cooled.
12. You'll need to stir more towards the end of the cooking, as you don't want the apple mixture to burn.
13. Once it's finished cooking, place in mason jars or another airtight container and store in the fridge.
14. Allow to cook for at least 3-4 hours.
15. Once cooled, you're ready to serve with toast.

Nutrition

- Calories: 1086kcal
- Carbohydrates: 291g
- Protein: 3g

- Fat: 2g

Lemon Crumb Cake with Lemon Curd

Servings: 12

Prep Time: 15 minutes

Cook Time: 45 minutes

Ingredients

Crumb topping:

- 3/4 cup blanched almond flour
- 1/4 cup organic refined coconut oil solid
- 1/4 cup + 2 Tbsp maple sugar coconut sugar will work too, but the color is much darker
- finely grated zest of one med lemon

Cake:

- 3 eggs room temp
- 1/4 cup fresh lemon juice about 2-3 lemons
- Grated zest of 1 medium lemon
- 3 Tbsp organic refined coconut oil melted and cooled to almost room temp
- 1 tsp pure vanilla extract
- 1/2 tsp pure almond extract
- 2/3 cup pure maple sugar coconut sugar will work too, the color will be much darker
- 2 cups blanched almond flour
- 1/3 cup tapioca flour
- 1/2 tsp baking soda
- 1/4 tsp salt
- 2/3 cup homemade lemon curd**

Icing:

- 2/3 cup organic powdered sugar Paleo option***
- 1 1/2 - 2 Tbsp lemon juice

Instructions

1. Preheat your oven to 350 degrees and line an 8 x 8" square baking pan with parchment paper on the bottom and sides, for easy removal.
2. Prepare the lemon curd, then set aside to cool to room temp while you prepare the cake.
3. Lemon curd can also be made ahead of time, if preferred.
4. Next, make the crumb topping by blending all ingredients with a fork or pastry blender until texture is crumbly, chill in the fridge while you prepare the cake batter.
5. In a large bowl, whisk together the eggs, lemon juice and zest, coconut oil, vanilla and almond extract, and sugar.

6. In a separate bowl, combine the almond flour, tapioca flour, baking soda, and salt.
7. Stir the dry mixture into the wet until well combined and smooth.
8. Using a silicone spatula, transfer cake batter into the parchment-lined cake pan and smooth out evenly.
9. Using a Tbsp, dollop the lemon curd over the cake batter, leaving 1/2" around the perimeter, then gently swirl with cake batter.
10. Sprinkle crumb topping all over the top to cover completely, then bake in the preheated oven for 35-40 mins until cake is set in the center.
11. Cool completely on a wire rack before slicing and serving.
12. For toppings, you can dust with organic powdered sugar (not paleo), drizzle on icing and garnish with grated lemon zest.
13. While cooling, prepare the icing/glaze of choice.
14. Whisk together ingredients until you get a consistency that you can drizzle (if making your powdered sugar, do this ahead of time) then use a spoon to drizzle icing over the cake as desired.
15. Enjoy!

Nutrition

- Calories: 316kcal
- Fat: 22g
- Carbohydrates: 24g
- Protein: 7g

Apple-Delicata Squash Porridge

Servings: 3

Prep Time: 10 mins

Cook Time: 18 mins

Total Time: 28 mins

Ingredients

- 4 small or 2 large apples unpeeled, flesh cut from the cores
- 1 delicata squash washed and whole
- 1/2 cup bone broth with little fat, or water instead
- 3 Tablespoons slippery elm optional for those on AIP
- 2 Tablespoons gelatin or up to 1/4 cup if eating the porridge hot (not chilled as pudding)
- 2 Tablespoons maple syrup, or honey for GAPS diet
- 1/2 teaspoon cinnamon
- 1/8 teaspoon each: cloves and ginger
- pinch sea salt

Instructions

1. Place whole, uncut delicata squash into instant pot.
2. Add apple chunks.
3. Add bone broth and spices.
4. Make sure rubber ring is in place in the Instant Pot lid, and secure lid, closing steam valve.
5. Choose Manual setting and 8 minutes.
6. When timer goes off, allow pressure to release naturally for 10 minutes; then press Cancel, place a dishtowel over steam valve and open it to release any remaining pressure.
7. Remove lid and insert, so the pot's contents begin to cool.
8. When cool enough to handle, place delicata on a plate or cutting board.
9. Cut in half length-wise and remove seeds with a spoon (They come out very quickly and easily).
10. Place squash halves and pot's contents (apples, broth, and spices) into a blender.
11. Add remaining ingredients: optional slippery elm, gelatin, maple syrup, and sea salt.
12. Blend for about 30 seconds, until smooth.
13. Serve with optional toppings, or pour into portable containers for packing in lunches.

Nutrition

- Calories 110
- Fat 1g
- Carbohydrates 22g
- Protein 7g

Instant Pot Quinoa Breakfast Bowls

Servings: 6

Prep Time: 25 minutes

Cook Time: 5 minutes

Total Time: 30 minutes

Ingredients

- 1 ½ cups quinoa, soaked for at least 1 hour
- 1 can coconut milk (or alternative milk)
- 1 ½ cups water
- 1 tsp ground cinnamon
- ¼ cup maple syrup
- ¼ teaspoon salt
- 2 tsp vanilla extract
- Fruit for toppings (optional)

Instructions

- Drain and rinse quinoa
- Place the quinoa, coconut milk, water, cinnamon, maple syrup, salt and vanilla in the Instant Pot
- Set to Rice setting and cook on low pressure for around 12 minutes
- Naturally release the pressure, then open the top and remove the lid
- Serve with any optional extras, and keep remaining mixture in the fridge for up to one week

Nutrition

- Calories: 197
- Carbohydrates: 36g
- Protein: 6g
- Fat: 2g

Easy Steel-Cut Oats

Servings: 4

Prep Time: 5 mins

Cook Time: 5 mins

Total Time: 10 mins

Ingredients

- 1 cup steel cut oats
- 3 cups water
- Fruit to mix in (optional)

Instructions

- Place steel cut oats and water into the Instant Pot
- Secure the lid and cook for 3 minutes
- When cooked, let pressure release naturally
- Stir in any fruit if desired, and serve

Nutrition

- Calories: 150
- Carbohydrates: 10g
- Protein: 7g
- Fat: 2.5g

Instant Pot Paleo Sweet Potato and Kale

Servings: 4

Prep Time: 10 mins

Cook Time: 20 mins

Total Time: 30 mins

Ingredients

- 1 tbsp olive oil
- ½ onion, diced
- ½ red pepper, diced
- 2 garlic cloves, minced
- 1 tsp chili powder
- 2 cups baby kale
- 1 ½ cups marinara sauce
- ½ teaspoon salt
- ½ teaspoon black pepper
- 2 sweet potatoes, boiled and chopped (keep these as mushed or firm as you like them)
- 1tbsp parsley, chopped
- ½ teaspoon smoked paprika
- ½ teaspoon ground cumin

Instructions

- Add olive oil, pepper, garlic, chili powder, paprika, cumin, pre-cooked sweet potato and onion to pot, and set on Saute function.
- Cook for around 3 minutes, until soft
- Add kale and cook for 2 minutes
- Add marinara sauce, salt and pepper
- Turn off pot and let cool
- Close lid and lock, and cook on low heat for 1 minute
- Quick-release pressure
- Serve sprinkled with parsley

Nutrition

- Calories: 123
- Carbohydrates: 9.8g
- Protein: 6.8g

- Fat: 8.2g

Instant Pot Breakfast Barley

Servings: 4

Prep Time: 10 minutes

Cook Time: 20 minutes

Cooling Time: 30 minutes

Ingredients

- 1 tbsp olive oil
- ¼ cup red onion, finely chopped
- 1 cup pearl barley
- 4 cups water or broth (or a mixture of the two)
- 1 teaspoon salt
- 4 ounces ham, diced
- 4 ounces baby kale

Instructions

- Set cooker to Manual, 18 minutes on the timer
- Add olive oil and heat
- Add barley and onion and heat for 3 minutes
- Add water, broth and salt, and close lid
- When the cooking is over, quick-release the pressure and drain most of the liquid
- Set the pot to Saute, then add the ham (if using)
- Stir occasionally
- Add the kale until wilted, then serve

Nutrition

- Calories: 217
- Carbohydrates: 15g
- Protein: 14g
- Fat: 10g

Easy Instant Pot Blueberry Jam

Servings: 3 jars

Prep Time: 5 mins

Cook Time: 2 hrs

Cooling Time: 3 hrs

Ingredients

- 5 cups blueberries (or other fruit of your choice)
- 1/2 cup honey

Instructions

- Add fruit and honey to inner pot
- Cook on low heat until honey melts, stirring occasionally
- When melted, turn up to high heat until pink and white bubbles showing
- Put the lid on the cooker and seal, and cook on High for 2 minutes
- Let pot depressurize naturally
- Remove lid, and cook on High until some water has boiled off and the jam is a nice, jammy consistency, stirring and scraping the bottom frequently
- Turn off cooker, and pour into jars

Nutrition

- Calories: 25
- Carbohydrates: 8g
- Protein: 1g
- Fat: 0.5g

Instant Pot Cinnamon Rolls

Servings: 8

Cook Time: 45 mins

Prep Time: 10 mins

Ingredients

For Dough:

- 1 cup blanched almond flour
- 1 1/2 cups arrowroot powder, plus more for dusting
- 1 t baking powder
- 1/4 t sea salt
- 1/3 cup warm water
- 3 T ghee, melted
- 2 t apple cider vinegar
- 1 large pasture-raised egg at room temperature

For Filling:

- 1/3 cup coconut sugar
- 1/4 cup cinnamon

Instructions

For the dough:

1. Gradually stir wet ingredients into the dry.
2. Add the egg and mix until combined.
3. Refrigerate for 15 minutes.
4. Line a cookie sheet with parchment paper and dust with arrowroot powder.
5. Press the dough into the cookie sheet, leaving a ¼" space around the edges.
   For the filling:

6. Mix the coconut sugar and cinnamon, then press the filling gently into the dough.
7. Freeze for 10 minutes.
8. Transfer to a working space and gently roll the dough off the parchment paper into a lengthwise log. Pinch both ends of the log to seal and slice into eight ½" rolls.
9. Grease a 7" push pan with ghee, and add the cinnamon rolls to the pushpan.
10. Cover with a paper towel and secure with a piece of aluminum foil on top.
11. Place the trivet inside the Instant Pot, add 2 cups of water, and set the pushpan with the rolls inside.
12. Lock the lid, secure the vent valve, and select Manual High for 20 minutes.

13. When the timer is done, allow the pressure to release before opening the vent valve and unlocking the lid.
14. Use the tongs to carefully remove the pan from the pot and slather Paleo frosting on top.

Nutrition

- Calories: 722
- Total Fat: 29g
- Carbohydrates: 103g
- Protein: 12g

AIP Tigernut Granola Recipe

Servings: 4

Prep Time: 5 minutes

Cook Time: 7 minutes

Ingredients

- 6 oz (165g) tigernuts
- 1 oz (30 g) coconut flakes
- 2 oz (60 g) mixed dried fruit
- 1 Tablespoon (15 ml) honey

Instructions

1. Preheat the oven to 350°F / 180°C.
2. Combine the tigernuts, coconut flakes, dried fruit, and honey in a bowl. Mix until well coated. Spread out in an even layer on a large roasting tray and place in the oven for 6-7 minutes. Remove the tray from the oven set aside to cool completely.
3. Serve with Greek yoghurt/dairy free yoghurt.
4. Store in a sealed container.

Nutrition

- Calories: 277
- Fat: 15 g Carbohydrates: 44 g
- Protein: 4 g

Apple Cranberry Crisp and Yoghurt In The Instant Pot

Servings: 4-6

Prep time: 20 minutes

Cook time: 20 minutes

Ingredients

For the filling:

- 3 medium apples, cored and cubed
- 2 firm pears, cored and cubed
- 1 1/2 cups cranberries (I used frozen)
- 1 tablespoon lemon juice
- 1/2 cup coconut sugar or sucanat or rapadura- feel free to increase if you prefer sweeter
- 2 tablespoons arrowroot powder
- 1/2 teaspoon ground ginger
- 1/4 teaspoon ground nutmeg
- 2 teaspoons ground cinnamon
- 1/2 teaspoon ground allspice
- 1/4 teaspoon ground cloves
- 1/4 teaspoon ground cardamom
- 1 teaspoon dried orange peel

For the topping:

- 1/2 cup coconut flour
- 1 tablespoon chia seeds
- 1 cup unsweetened shredded coconut
- 1/2 cup walnuts or pecans; soak and dehydrate your own!
- 1/4 cup coconut sugar or sucanat or rapadura
- 1 teaspoon ground cinnamon
- 1 pinch ground nutmeg
- 1/4 teaspoon sea salt
- 1/2 cup coconut oil or butter, softened but not melted

Instructions

To make the filling:

1. Combine cored and cubed apples and pears in the bottom of an 8-inch, 2-quart oven-safe dish, such as this one.
2. Then add cranberries, lemon juice, sweetener, arrowroot powder, and spices.
3. Mix until evenly distributed.

To make the topping:

1. In a separate, small mixing bowl, combine coconut flour, chia seeds, coconut, nuts if desired, sweetener, spices, and salt.
2. Add coconut oil in small chunks.
3. Then mix gently with a fork until evenly distributed.

To make the apple cranberry crisp:

1. Layer topping over filling ingredients.
2. Make a foil sling to go under the baking dish. And make sure to reinforce your sling with extra pieces of aluminum foil, as this dish becomes too heavy for a single piece of aluminum folded lengthwise.
3. Add 2 cups of water and a trivet to pressure cooker.
4. Then, using the foil sling to transport, gently lower the baking dish inside the cooker.
5. Put on the lid of your cooker, checking that the seals and all components are in good shape, including being in the sealed position.
6. If using an electric cooker, set to high for 20 minutes.
7. If using a stove-top cooker, bring to high pressure and maintain pressure for a cook time of 20 minutes.
8. Once the cycle is complete, if using an electric cooker, hit the Cancel button to turn off the heat.
9. With a stove-top cooker, remove from heat.
10. Then place a towel over the pressure release knob and allow the pot to do a quick pressure release.
11. When pressure is released, open lid.
12. Carefully remove crisp from the cooker using foil sling.
13. For a crisper, crunchier top, place under the broiler in the oven for a few minutes until browned.
14. Then serve with a dollop of Greek yoghurt.

Nutrition

- Calories: 185
- Total Fat: 4.9g
- Carbohydrates: 31.6g
- Protein: 5.3g

Chapter 6: Snack & Bites Recipes

AIP Raw Brownie Bites

Servings: 1 Brownie Bite Portion (Makes 24 mini bites)

Prep Time: 10 mins

Cook Time: nil (requires 20 mins chilling time)

Total Time: 20 mins

Ingredients

- 14 oz (400 g) soft dates
- 3 tablespoons (18 g) carob powder
- 3 tablespoons (45 ml) coconut oil, melted but not too hot
- 1/4 cup (20 g) unsweetened shredded coconut

Instructions

1. Place the dates, carob powder, and melted coconut oil into a mini food processor and blitz until completely combined. Scrape the mass out onto a tray lined with parchment paper and use the back of a metal spoon to flatten the mixture into a large, compact square approx. 3/4-inch high.
2. Scatter over the shredded coconut and use clean hands to 'press' the coconut gently onto the surface.
3. Place the tray into the fridge for about 20 minutes, then slice into small 1-inch squares.
4. Store covered in the fridge.

Nutrition

- Calories: 70
- Fat: 2 g
- Carbohydrates: 14 g
- Protein: 0 g

AIP Baked Pita Chips

Servings: 2

Prep Time: 5 mins

Cook Time: 20 mins

Total Time: 25 mins

Ingredients

- 1/3 cup (43 g) arrowroot
- 1/3 cup (40 g) tapioca or cassava flour
- 3 tablespoons (45 ml) olive oil
- 4 tablespoons (60 ml) cold water

Instructions

1. Preheat oven to 400 F (200 C).
2. Mix all the ingredients well with your hands.
3. Place on a piece of parchment paper and roll flat (approx. 2mm-thick).
4. Score the dough to form small 1-inch squares.
5. Place in oven and bake for 15-20 minutes (check to make sure it doesn't burn).
6. Remove and cool before enjoying.

Nutrition

- Calories: 160
- Fat: 11 g
- Protein: 0 g

AIP Tigernut Granola

Servings: 4

Prep Time: 5 mins

Cook Time: 7 mins

Total Time: 12 mins

Ingredients

- 6 oz (165g) tigernuts
- 1 oz (30 g) coconut flakes
- 2 oz (60 g) mixed dried fruit
- 1 tablespoon (15 ml) honey

Instructions

5. Preheat the oven to 350°F / 180°C.
6. Combine the tigernuts, coconut flakes, dried fruit, and honey in a bowl. Mix until well coated. Spread out in an even layer on a large roasting tray and place in the oven for 6-7 minutes. Remove the tray from the oven set aside to cool completely.
7. Store in a sealed container.

Nutrition

- Calories: 277
- Fat: 15 g Carbohydrates: 44 g
- Protein: 4 g

AIP Nori Bites

Servings: 8 bites (2 Servings)

Prep Time: 15 mins

Cook Time: nil

Total Time: 15 mins

Ingredients

For the sauce:

- 3 tablespoons (45 ml) of coconut cream
- 1 teaspoon (5 ml) of coconut aminos

For the nori bites:

- 2 nori sheets
- 5.3 oz of smoked salmon (148 g)
- 1/4 cucumber (55 g), cut into thin sticks
- 1/4 carrot (13 g), peeled and sliced into matchsticks
- 1 green onion (5 g), sliced
- cilantro, to garnish

Instructions

1. Make sauce by combining the coconut cream and coconut aminos. Set aside.
2. Cut the nori sheets into 4 equal pieces to create 8 little squares.
3. Dampen the nori by running a damp finger over the sheets until they can roll up.
4. Place a small dollop of sauce onto each square then add the rest of the ingredients onto each piece.
5. Roll up the squares and enjoy!

Nutrition

- Calories: 152
- Fat: 7 g
- Carbohydrates: 3 g
- Protein: 15 g

Cassava Fries Instant Pot {Paleo, AIP}

Servings: 4

Prep Time: 15 mins

Cook Time: 1 hr 25 mins

Total Time: 1 hr 45 mins

Ingredients

- 2 pounds cassava root, frozen or fresh
- 2 cups filtered water
- 3/4 cup fat (duck fat is best), then lard, then Kerrygold butter, then strained bacon fat, then coconut oil or avocado oil, then tallow
- 1 teaspoon sea salt garnish

Instructions

1. Place water into base of Instant Pot insert.
2. Add cassava root.
3. Check that rubber ring is fitted inside Instant Pot lid.
4. Place lid on Instant Pot, making sure the steam release valve is sealed.
5. Press the "Manual" setting, and decrease the time until you reach 25 minutes.
6. When the Instant Pot is done and beeps, press "Cancel."
7. Allow Instant Pot to release pressure naturally for 30 minutes.
8. Place a dish towel or oven mitt over the steam valve, and open it to release any remaining pressure.
9. Remove lid and insert, so the pot's contents begin to cool.
10. Cool cassava almost completely; then transfer to a cutting surface.
11. The roots will have split open during cooking, or they will easily splay open.
12. Remove tough, stringy fiber that runs down the center of each one.
13. Slice roots into long strips of desired thickness; about 8 fries per root. Cassava-fries-instruction
14. Place fat in heavy bottom pot over high heat
15. When fat is quite hot (sizzles when a drop of water is added) carefully add cassava strips in rows.
16. Cook cassava on first side about 5 minutes, then reduce heat to medium-high or medium
17. Flip each strip over, using two forks or a set of tongs.
18. Remove cassava fries to a large plate
19. Serve fries with extra sea salt and any optional dippings you like.

Nutrition

- Calories 702
- Fat 351

- Carbohydrates 86g
- Protein 3g

Chapter 7: Soup & Salad Recipes

Paleo Egg Roll Soup (Whole30, AIP)

Servings: 5

Prep time: 10 mins

Cook time: 30 mins

Total time: 40 mins

Ingredients

- 1 lb ground pork (see above for substitutions)
- 2 tbsp coconut oil (sub sesame oil for non-AIP/if tolerated)
- 1 white onion, diced
- 1 cup carrots, shredded
- 1 small green cabbage, sliced into strips
- 6 cups chicken broth
- 1 tbsp coconut aminos
- 1 tsp garlic powder
- 1 tsp ginger powder
- 1/2 –1 tsp sea salt
- 2 tbsp green onion, chopped
- Optional- Sriracha to taste (omit for AIP)

Instructions

1. Using a large pot, brown the ground pork on medium heat and lightly salt.
2. Set aside when cooked and discard the fat.
3. Melt the coconut oil in the pot on medium heat and add the diced onion.
4. Saute for 5 minutes or until lightly translucent.
5. Add the carrot and gently sauté for a few minutes until the carrots soften slightly.
6. Pour in the broth, cabbage, cooked pork, coconut aminos, garlic powder, and grated ginger, and mix well to combine.
7. Bring the soup to a low simmer and cook for 15-20 minutes or until the cabbage is wilted.
8. Season further to taste and top the soup with sliced green onion to serve

Nutrition

- Calories: 336
- Fat: 24.8g
- Carbohydrates: 7.5g
- Protein: 20.4g

Chicken Drumstick Soup

Servings: 6

Prep Time: 15 minutes

Cook Time: 35 minutes

Total Time: 50 minutes

Ingredients

- 1 1/2 pounds chicken drumsticks - about five large ones
- 2 large ribs celery, sliced
- 2 medium carrots, peeled and diced
- 1 large parsnip, peeled and diced
- 1 medium rutabaga, peeled and diced
- 1 small yellow onion, diced
- 2 bay leaves
- 1/2 teaspoon cracked black pepper
- 1-quart chicken broth or 1-quart water + 1 teaspoon salt

Instructions

1. Layer all of the ingredients in the pot, pouring in the chicken broth last to avoid splashing.
2. Cover the pot and set it to "Soup" setting. Wait for the program to finish and pot to depressurize.
3. When you can safely open the pot, remove the drumsticks with a slotted spoon and allow them to rest just until cool enough to handle.
4. Remove the meat from the drumsticks, discarding the bones, skin, and cartilage. Return the meat to the pot with the other ingredients.
5. Check for seasoning and salt to taste, if desired. Ladle into bowls and serve.

Nutrition

- Calories: 150
- Fat: 5g
- Carbohydrate: 0g
- Protein: 15g

Instant Pot AIP Paleo Chicken Fennel Soup

Servings: 6-8

Prep Time: 20 mins

Cook Time: 30 mins

Total Time: 50 mins

Ingredients

- 1 pound boneless, skinless chicken breast or/and thighs, cut into chunks
- 1 large bulb fennel, chopped
- 1/2 onion, chopped
- 4 green onions, chopped
- 1 cup chopped kale or spinach
- 3 cloves garlic, peeled and chopped
- 2 cups chicken or bone broth
- 4 cups of filtered water
- 1 bay leaf
- 1 tablespoon dried oregano
- 1/8 teaspoon salt

Instructions

1. Add all ingredients to Instant Pot.
2. Place lid on the pot.
3. Press the Soup button. (Be sure it's set to 30 minutes cook time)
4. When cooking has stopped, allow the pot to release pressure naturally for 10 minutes.
5. Open lid.
6. Serve.

Nutrition

- Calories:246
- Fat: 10g
- Carbohydrate: 33g
- Protein: 6g

Quick Onion Soup {AIP}

Servings: 6

Prep Time: 30 minutes

Cook Time: 35 minutes

Total Time: 1 hour 5 minutes

Ingredients

- 2 tbsp / 30 ml avocado oil, coconut oil or good quality lard
- 8 cups / 960 g yellow onions
- 1 tbsp / 15 ml balsamic vinegar
- 6 cups / 1.4 L pork stock
- 1 tsp / 5 g real salt
- 2 bay leaves
- 2 large sprigs of fresh thyme

Instructions

1. Cut the onions in half through the root, peel them and slice them into thin half-moons.
2. Set the Instant Pot to "Saute" and add the oil.
3. Once the oil is hot, add the onions.
4. Cook the onions until they have reduced down and become translucent, stirring occasionally to prevent sticking; about 15 minutes.
5. Add the balsamic vinegar and scrape up any food from the bottom of the Instant Pot, then add the stock, salt, bay leaves and thyme.
6. Turn off the Instant Pot and close the lid of the Instant Pot, making sure to check that the float is free and the vent isn't blocked and that the lid is set in the "Sealing" position.
7. Set the Instant Pot to "High Pressure" and cook the soup for 10 minutes once it has come up to pressure. Allow the pressure to release using the "natural release" – don't open the vent or hot liquid may gush out of the vent along with the steam.
8. Discard the bay leaves and thyme stems, then blend the soup either using an immersion blender directly in the pot or by transferring the soup carefully to a blender.

Nutrition

- Calories:290
- Fat: 9.6g
- Carbohydrate: 33.4g
- Protein: 16.8g

Split Asparagus Soup

Serving: 4-6

Prep Time: 10 minutes

Cook Time: 20 minutes

Total Time: 30 minutes

Ingredients

- 2 lb asparagus, split (i.e. chopped in half)
- 3 tbsp ghee
- 5 cloves garlic, pressed
- 1 white onion, diced
- 1 ham bone (or 1 C diced ham)
- 4 C chicken broth
- 1/2 tsp dried thyme
- salt and pepper to taste

Instructions

1. Set your Instant Pot to Sauté, and melt your ghee.
2. Add diced onions, and cook for approximately 5 minutes, or until the onion starts to brown.
3. Add in pressed garlic, ham bone, and broth, and simmer for 2-3 minutes.
4. Place in your thyme and asparagus and seal the Instant Pot. Set to Soup setting and adjust the time to 45 minutes.
5. Allow to vent, blend with a food processor, and serve!

Nutrition

- Calories: 181.5kcal
- Fat: 6g
- Carbohydrate: 18g
- Protein: 4g

Instant Pot (Pressure Cooker) Bo Kho (Vietnamese Beef Stew)

Servings: 8

Prep Time: 5 mins

Cook Time: 1 hr 10 mins

Total Time: 1 hr 25 mins

Ingredients

- ½ teaspoon ghee
- 5 pounds bone-in short ribs OR 2½ pounds grass-fed beef brisket or chuck roast trimmed and cut into 1½-inch cubes (all work equally well)
- 1 yellow onion, peeled and diced
- 1½ teaspoons, Madras curry powder
- 2½ tablespoons, peeled and microplaned fresh ginger
- 2 cups canned diced tomatoes, drained and crushed by hand
- 3 tablespoons Red Boat fish sauce
- 2 tablespoons applesauce
- 1 large stalk lemongrass trimmed of loose leaves, cut into 3-inch lengths, and bruised with a heavy object (e.g. ramekin, meat pounder, the broad side of a kitchen knife—you get the idea)
- 2 whole star anise
- 1 bay leaf
- 1 cup bone broth
- 1 pound carrots, peeled and chopped into 1-inch pieces
- Kosher salt

Instructions

1. Grab your pressure cooker and melt the ghee over medium-high heat. If you have an Instant Pot, use the "Sauté" function to heat the fat. Dry off the ribs and sear them in the pressure cooker.
2. Fry the beef in batches because you don't want to overcrowd them in the pressure cooker. Transfer the seared beef to a separate bowl or plate.
3. Toss in the onions and sauté until translucent.
4. Add the curry powder, ginger, seared beef, diced tomatoes, fish sauce, applesauce, star anise, smashed lemongrass stalks, and bay leaf. Pour in the broth.
5. Cover and lock the lid of your pressure cooker.
6. If you're using an Instant Pot, press the clear/off button before pressing the "Manual" or "Pressure Cook" button. Program the Instant Pot to cook for 50 minutes under high pressure. (If you're using cubed brisket or chuck roast, set it to cook for 35 minutes under high pressure.) Once the pot is programmed, walk away.

7. Using a stove-top pressure cooker? You won't have all those buttons to press; instead, just cook covered on high heat until high pressure is reached. Then, reduce the heat to low to maintain high pressure for about 45 minutes if you're cooking short ribs, and 30 minutes if you're cooking cubed brisket or chuck roast.

8. When the stew is finished cooking, turn off the pressure cooker. Turn the valve at the top of the lid to release the pressure immediately.

9. Once the pressure's dropped, pop open the lid and add the carrots. Cook for 7 minutes under high pressure.

10. This time, when the stew finishes cooking, turn off the pressure cooker and let the pressure drop naturally. If the pressure hasn't dropped completely after 15 minutes, turn the valve at the top of the lid to fully release the pressure.

11. Adjust the stew for seasoning with salt and fish sauce if needed.

12. Dig in right away—or store the stew in the fridge or freezer to eat at a later date. The stew will keep in an airtight container for up to 4 days in the fridge and several months in the freezer.

Nutrition

- Calories: 494
- Carbohydrates: 11g
- Protein: 61g
- Fat: 22g

Instant Pot Beef Stew with Turnips and Carrots

Servings: 4

Prep time: 15 mins

Cook time: 60 mins

Total time: 1 hr 15 mins

Ingredients

- 1 pound beef stew meat, preferably grass-fed, cut into 1 inch pieces salt
- 2 tablespoons cooking fat of choice (I used bacon grease, but lard, tallow, or coconut oil would also work well)
- 1 medium red onion, chopped
- 2 tablespoons cassava flour
- 1 teaspoon dried thyme
- 1 cup dry red wine
- 1 cup bone broth, preferably homemade
- 1 pound turnips, cut into 1 inch pieces
- 1 pound carrots, cut into 1 inch pieces
- ¼ cup coconut aminos
- ¼ cup chopped fresh parsley

Instructions

1. Season beef with salt.
2. Plugin Instant Pot and press the Sauté button.
3. Once heated, put 1 tablespoon of fat in to melt.
4. Add beef and brown on all sides (should take about 8 minutes total).
5. Remove beef and set aside.
6. Add remaining fat and onions to Instant Pot and cook, stirring constantly, until soft (about 5 minutes).
7. Stir in cassava flour and thyme and cook for about one minute.
8. Whisk in wine, scraping up any browned bits on the bottom of the pot.
9. Stir in broth, turnips, carrots, coconut aminos, and reserved beef.
10. Place lid on Instant Pot and lock it into place.
11. Press the "Meat/Stew" button.
12. When cooking is complete, allow pressure to release naturally for about 10 minutes, then quickly release any remaining pressure.
13. Ladle into individual bowls and garnish with parsley.

Nutrition

- Calories: 302

- Fat: 7g
- Carbohydrate: 26g
- Protein: 35g

Paleo Chicken & Smoked Sausage Stew

Servings: 6

Prep Time: 15 minutes

Cook Time: 25 minutes

Total Time: 40 minutes

Ingredients:

- 1 pound boneless, skinless chicken thighs
- 1 pound andouille pork sausage
- 1 tablespoon coconut oil
- 6 cups chopped tomatoes
- 1 medium white onion
- 2 stalks celery
- 2 large carrots
- 2 cups bone broth or water
- 1/4 cup parsley
- 6 cloves garlic
- 1 teaspoon sea salt
- 1 teaspoon thyme
- 1/2 teaspoon smoked paprika
- 1/2 teaspoon crushed red chili flakes
- 1/4 teaspoon black pepper
- 1/4 teaspoon cayenne
- 1 bay leaf
- Optional: hot sauce to taste

Instructions

1. Heat the coconut oil in the bottom of the Instant Pot (on the Sauté setting). Add the chicken and sausage to the pan and cook through (about 4-5 minutes on each side). While the meat cooks, slice the onion. Dice the bell peppers, and chop the carrots and celery. Remove the meat from the pot, and set aside for later use.
2. Sauté the vegetables in the bottom of the Instant Pot, stirring occasionally. Mince the garlic, and add it to the pan. Add the broth and chopped tomatoes. Bring the mixture to a simmer (the sauté function will do this automatically)
3. Once the chicken and sausage are cool enough to handle, slice them into bite-sized pieces. Return them to the pot, along with the spices. Mince the parsley now, and add that as well. Give the stew one stir and then lock the lid on. Turn the Instant Pot to the soup setting and cook for 5-10 minutes.

4. Serve warm with hot sauce to taste. Note: This recipe can be done in a regular soup pot; just increase the final cooking time in step 3 to 20 to 30 minutes, until the vegetables are tender and the flavors have simmered together.

Nutrition

- Calories: 268
- Fat: 18g
- Carbohydrate: 10g
- Protein: 13g

Pressure Cooker Beet & Caper Salad

Servings: 2

Prep time: 5 mins

Cook time: 30 mins

Total time: 35 mins

Ingredients

- 4 medium beets
- 2 tablespoons white balsamic vinegar (or rice wine vinegar)

Dressing:

- A small bunch of parsley stems removed (about 1 heaping tablespoon, chopped)
- 1 large garlic clove
- ½ teaspoon salt
- 1 pinch black pepper
- 1 tablespoon extra virgin olive oil
- 2 tablespoons capers

Instructions

1. Prepare the pressure cooker by adding one cup of water and the steamer basket and set aside.
2. Snip the tops of the beets and clean well - taking care not to pierce the skin.
3. Put the beets in the steamer basket.
4. Close and lock the lid of the pressure cooker. For stovetop pressure cookers, turn the heat up to high and when the cooker reaches pressure, lower to the heat to the minimum required by the cooker to maintain pressure. Cook for 20-25 minutes at high pressure.
5. In the meantime, prepare the dressing by chopping garlic and parsley together and then putting in a small jar with the salt, pepper, olive oil, and capers. Close tightly and shake vigorously.
6. When time is up, open the cooker by releasing the pressure.
7. Check beets for doneness: a fork should easily pierce through to the center. If it does not, pop the lid back onto the pressure cooker and cook for 5 more minutes at high pressure with Normal pressure release.
8. Move the steamer basket to the sink and run cold water over the beets to cool. Then, using your fingers (optionally wearing gloves) or a dull knife, brush the skin off.
9. If your sink/cutting board configuration allows, place a plastic cutting board in the sink (to prevent beet juice splatters and spills) and slice beets.
10. Arrange on serving platter and sprinkle with vinegar - store this way tightly covered to serve up to four days later - give the dressing a final shake and pour onto the beets just before serving.

Nutrition

- Calories: 43.1
- Fat: 2.4g
- Carbohydrate: 5.4g
- Protein: 0.7g

Creamed Fennel and Cauliflower Soup

Servings: 4

Prep Time: 5 minutes

Cook Time: 25 minutes

Total Time: 30 mins

Ingredients:

For the salad:

- 1 tablespoon coconut oil
- 1 white onion
- 3 cloves garlic
- 1 extra-large or 2 medium-sized fennel bulbs, stalks and fronds removed
- 1 pound cauliflower florets
- 1 cup coconut milk
- 3 cups broth (bone broth or vegetable broth)
- 2 teaspoons salt
- Optional: Truffle oil, for serving
- Optional: Black pepper for serving (NOTE: this recipe is AIP-friendly if you skip the pepper).

Instructions

1. Slice the onions, mince the garlic, and chop the fennel.
2. If your cauliflower is not already chopped into florets, do that now.
3. At the bottom of your pressure cooker, heat up the coconut oil.
4. Sauté the onions until translucent.
5. Add the garlic, fennel, and cauliflower.
6. Sauté for 5-10 minutes, until the edges of the vegetables begin to turn golden.
7. Pour the broth and coconut milk into the pot.
8. Add salt. Cook on the soup setting for at least 5 minutes.
9. Once the pressure cooker is done cooking, release the pressure and remove the lid.
10. Use a standing blender or an immersion blender to puree the soup to a smooth, creamy consistency.
11. Scoop into serving bowls and drizzle with truffle oil.
12. Top with freshly cracked pepper, and garnish with a leftover fennel frond.
13. Serve hot.

Nutrition

- Calories: 168
- Fat: 12.2g
- Carbohydrate: 11.4g

- Protein: 4.5g

Easy Instant Pot Sweet Potato & Beef Stew (AIP, Paleo)

Servings: 4

Prep Time: 20 minutes

Cook Time: 1 hour

Total Time: 1 hour 20 minutes

Ingredients

- 1 tsp avocado oil
- 1 onion diced
- 1 tbsp ginger minced, or 1 tsp dried
- 3 cloves garlic minced, or 2 tsp dried
- 1 cup carrots, sliced into large chunks
- 5 cups sweet potatoes, peeled and cubed
- 2 tsp dried oregano or 2 tbsp fresh
- 2 tsp dried thyme or 2 tbsp fresh
- 1 tsp sea salt
- 1 1/2 tsp freshly ground black pepper - optional
- 1 cup pumpkin puree
- 2 cups bone broth
- 1 lb ground beef, grass-fed if possible
- juice of 1 lemon or 2 limes
- 1 cup cilantro or parsley, chopped
- 6 green onions, sliced
- Avocado, diced

Instructions

1. Set Instant Pot to "sauté" function and heat avocado oil.
2. When the oil is hot, add onion, ginger, garlic, carrots, sweet potatoes, oregano, thyme, sea salt, and black pepper, and sauté for a few minutes until fragrant.
3. Turn Instant Pot off, and add pumpkin puree and bone broth. Stir to combine.
4. Add ground beef to insert in a single layer.
5. Using the manual setting, cook stew on high pressure for 5 minutes.
6. Use the quick-release method to release pressure when the stew is done cooking.
7. Stir in lemon juice and taste for seasoning. Divide among four bowls.
8. Top with fresh herbs and avocado to serve.

Nutrition

- Calories: 394.9
- Fat: 20.2g
- Carbohydrate: 24g
- Protein: 28.3g

Instant Pot Popeye Soup (Paleo, AIP)

Servings:

Prep Time: 5 mins

Cook Time: 15 mins

Total Time: 20 mins

Ingredients

- 2 tablespoons ghee
- 1 large onion, coarsely chopped
- 1 large head of cauliflower, coarsely chopped (florets only)
- 2 ounces (1 bunch) cilantro
- 12 ounces (1 head) broccoli, coarsely chopped (about 2 cups)
- 3 ounces baby spinach leaves
- 5 cups chicken broth
- 1 cup coconut milk (or an extra cup of broth)
- 1 tablespoon garlic, chopped
- 1 tablespoon of sea salt
- 2 teaspoons onion powder
- Black pepper to taste (omit for AIP)
- optional: shredded chicken from one rotisserie chicken or sauteed mushrooms to top/mix in

Instructions

1- Spoon the ghee into the stainless steel bowl of your Instant Pot and press the "Saute" button
2- Introduce the onion to the ghee and sauté for 10 minutes, stirring occasionally so the onion does not burn (note from Amanda: this step is optional if you are pressed for time! But it does add flavor to the soup).
3- Now place all remaining ingredients into the bowl, press the "Keep Warm/Cancel" button, and secure the lid.
4- Now close off the pressure valve and then press the "Manual" button.
5- Adjust the time with the "-" button until it reads 5 minutes (note from Amanda: I only cook veggies for 3 minutes and it always works great for me!).
6- Allow the cooking cycle to complete and then release the pressure valve.
7- Remove the lid when safe to do so and then use an immersion blender to completely puree all ingredients.
8- The soup should be thick and creamy. If you want it thinner, you can add more broth until the desired consistency is reached.
9- Serve topped with fresh herbs if desired (note from Amanda: I stirred in shredded chicken from 1 whole bird to make it a complete meal. I also served some topped with sauteed shiitake and lion's mane mushrooms and it was fab!).

Nutrition

- Calories: 50
- Fat: 0g
- Carbohydrate: 0g
- Protein: 4g

Ugly Soup (AIP, Paleo)

Servings: 8

Prep time: 20 mins

Cooking time: 15 mins

Total Time: 35 mins

Ingredients

- 1 lb ground turkey
- 1 1/2 roughly chopped carrots
- 2 1/2 diced white sweet potatoes
- 1 cup sliced red onion
- 3 cups kale, loosely packed, chopped, stems removed
- 2 TBSP apple cider vinegar
- 1 1/2 tsp sea salt*
- 1 sprig fresh rosemary
- 4-6 sprigs fresh thyme
- 6 cups bone broth

Instructions

1- Crumble turkey on the bottom of the bowl of a pressure cooker. Add everything else in order.
2- Pressure cook at 10.5 psi, then auto release for 15 minutes. Remove herb sprigs. Stir and serve!

Nutrition

- Calories: 136
- Fat: 4g
- Carbohydrate: 4g
- Protein: 19g

Creamy Goat Stew with Taro

Servings: 4

Prep Time: 10 minutes

Cook Time: 35 minutes

Total Time: 45 minutes

Ingredients

- 2 cups/ 300g taro/ eddoes, cut into 1 inch chunks
- Avocado oil/ animal fat (enough to form a layer in a heavy-bottomed pot)
- 1 small onion, peeled and chopped
- 1 tbsp coconut oil
- 1lb/ 500g young goat meat, cubed into 1 inch cubes
- 1 cup bone broth
- 4 cloves garlic, smashed
- 1 leek, white part cut into ½ inch rings or 3 green onions, cut into 1 inch long pieces
- 1 cup coconut milk
- Sea salt, to taste
- 1 tbsp coriander leaves, chopped

Instructions

1. Fry the taro/ eddo chunks in a layer of hot oil/fat in a heavy-bottomed pot over medium heat until crisp.
2. Drain over kitchen paper towels and set aside.
3. Using the Sauté function, cook the onion in 1 tbsp coconut oil until translucent.
4. Remove and set aside.
5. Working in batches, brown the goat meat in the pressure cooker pot until seared on all sides.
6. Top up with extra oil if necessary.
7. Set aside.
8. Pour the bone broth into the pot, stirring gently to remove any browned bits of meat stuck to the bottom of the pot.
9. Add in the onions, browned meat, garlic and leeks or green onions.
10. Cover the pot with the pressure cooker lid and set the valve to 'sealing'.
11. Cook for 20 minutes under 'Manual' setting.
12. Once the cooking time is completed, press 'cancel' and allow the cooker to cool naturally until the pressure is released.
13. You may speed up the pressure release duration by placing damp, cool towels on the lid.
14. Select the 'Saute' function and add in the cooked taro chunks and coconut milk, stirring gently to mix. Add sea salt to taste.

15. Let it simmer until the taro chunks are cooked and gravy thickened slightly. This should not take more than 5 minutes.

    .

16. Sprinkle with chopped coriander.
17. Enjoy!

Nutrition

- Calories: 477.2
- Fat: 18.1g
- Carbohydrate: 51.2g
- Protein: 30.2g

Low FODMAP Beef Stew (AIP, Paleo, Whole 30)

Servings: 6-8

Prep Time: 15 minutes

Cook Time: 8 hours

Total Time: 8 hours 15 minutes

Ingredients

- 2 tbsp solid fat
- 2 lbs grassfed beef Stew meat
- 4 strips bacon, cut into small pieces
- 2 heaping cups (approximately 140 g) chopped leek greens and/or scallion greens
- 2 heaping cups (approximately 425 g) chopped carrots
- 2 heaping cups (approximately 365 g) cubed rutabaga
- 1.5 c bone broth
- 1.5 c red wine (I've used both Merlot and Cabernet Sauvignon)
- 2 dried bay leaves
- 1 tbsp salt
- Few sprigs of fresh thyme & parsley, plus additional for serving

Instructions

1. Add the fat to the insert of an Instant Pot.
2. Turn the pot onto "Sauté" & allow the fat to melt.
3. Dry the meat very well. Brown the beef on all sides, in batches, in the sautéing Instant Pot
4. Remove the browned beef & set aside.
5. Sauté the bacon & leek/scallion greens in the Instant Pot until the bacon begins to crisp & the leeks/scallions begin to wilt. Stir occasionally.
6. Add the carrots & rutabaga, broth, wine, and browned beef. Stir to combine.
7. Tuck the bay leaf & herbs into the mixture.
8. Place the top on the Instant Pot & make sure the vent is closed.
9. Pressure cook using the manual setting for 50 minutes at high heat.
10. Note: the entire process will take longer than 50 minutes because it does take time for the pot to come up to pressure.
11. Once the machine has beeped, allow it to switch to the "keep warm" function or turn completely off for 15 minutes to let the pressure come down a bit.
12. Use a silicone oven mitt or heavy kitchen towel to move the vent from the "sealing" position to the "venting" position.
13. Allow all the steam to escape then it is safe to open the lid.
14. Serve the stew on its own, or alongside a starchy vegetable.
15. Adding extra cooked greens is also a great option.

16. Sprinkle with some extra chopped herbs just before serving.
17. Store any leftovers in the refrigerator or freezer.

Nutrition

- Calories: 302
- Fat: 7g
- Carbohydrate: 26g
- Protein: 35g

Chapter 8: Vegetable Recipes

Instant Pot Smothered Cajun Greens

Servings: 4

Prep Time: 15 mins

Cook Time: 20 mins

Total Time: 35 mins

Ingredients

- 6 cups raw greens (collard, mustard, turnip, spinach, kale, etc.)
- 1 turnip, chopped
- 1 onion, chopped
- 1 pound fully cooked, uncured ham, cut into large chunks
- 1 tablespoon animal fat (I used bacon fat)
- 2 teaspoons (about 2 cloves) crushed garlic
- 1/8 teaspoon salt
- 1/2 cup poultry broth (bone broth, if you have it)

Instructions

1. Place all ingredients into Instant Pot and Close lid.
2. Press the Manual button and set to 20 minute cook time.
3. Press the Pressure button to set on high pressure.
4. When done cooking, turn off Instant Pot.
5. Allow pressure to reduce naturally for 10 minutes.
6. Turn the pressure valve to Venting.
7. Open the lid once all pressure is released.
8. Stir.
9. Serve.

Nutrition

- Calories: 80
- Fat: 2g
- Carbohydrate: 15g
- Protein: 6g

Instant Pot Spaghetti Squash with Duck Fat Apple Juice Glaze

Servings: 6

Prep time: 15 minutes

Cook Time: 25 minutes

Total Time: 40 minutes

Ingredients

- 1 spaghetti squash (around 3 lbs)
- 3/4 cup apple juice
- 2 tbsp. duck fat
- Real salt, to taste

Instructions

1. Put the rack that came with your Instant Pot in the bottom of the stainless steel insert.
2. Pour 1 cup water over it, and set spaghetti squash (whole) on top of the rack.
3. Close and lock the lid.
4. You'll see the display light up to indicate high pressure 30 minutes.
5. Wait 5 seconds, and the pot will beep and the display will say ON.
6. This means it's heating up and building up pressure, which takes about 11 minutes.
7. Once full pressure is reached, the display will switch and start counting down the cooking time (20 minutes).
8. The Instant Pot will beep when the 20 minutes are up.
9. Carefully turn the pressure knob to the "Venting" position.
10. Once all the steam is released, you can open the pot.
11. Use hot pads to lift the squash out of the pot and set it on a cutting board.
12. Cut it in half, and let it start to cool off.
13. Remove the rack and empty the water.
14. Put the stainless steel insert back into pot.
15. Now it's time to make the sauce in the Instant Pot.
16. Pour the apple juice into the stainless steel insert, and click the "Sauté" button.
17. The display will again light up saying 30 and beneath it, the "Normal" light will be lit. Click the "Adjust" button until the display switches from "Normal" to "More."
18. Wait a few seconds, and the main display will switch to "On". Within a few minutes, the juice will start simmering.
19. Let it simmer for about 3 minutes to reduce the liquid and concentrate the flavor. Then add the duck fat and stir until melted. Click the "Cancel" button to turn off the Instant Pot.
20. Scoop out the seeds from the spaghetti squash and throw them away. Then, use a fork to scrape the spaghetti squash noodles into the pot.

21. Season generously with sea salt, and toss to coat evenly with the glaze.
22. Taste, and add more salt if needed.

Nutrition

- Calories: 42
- Fat: 0.5g
- Carbohydrate: 10g
- Protein: 1g

Lemon - Garlic Hummus (AIP, Paleo, Instant Pot)

Servings: 1 ¾ cup per person

Prep time: 10 mins

Cook time: 10 mins

Total time: 20 mins

Ingredients

- 1 cup water
- 1 medium sweet potato, cut in half lengthwise (about 1/2 pound)
- 1 medium turnip, cut in half lengthwise (about 1/2 pound)
- 1 head garlic
- 3 tablespoons extra-virgin olive oil
- 2 tablespoons coconut milk
- 2 tablespoons lemon juice
- 1 teaspoon onion powder
- 1/2 teaspoon sea salt, or more to taste

Instructions

1. Pour water into the Instant Pot and add the steamer rack. Place sweet potatoes, turnips, and garlic on the steamer rack.
2. Close and lock the lid. Press MANUAL for High pressure. Set cooking time to 10 minutes. Once time is up, allow the pressure to release naturally.
3. If you don't have an Instant Pot, you can simply steam the vegetables and garlic or roast them in the oven.
4. Let vegetables cool down completely before peeling.
5. In a high-speed blender, add peeled vegetables, peeled garlic, and all the other ingredients. Mix on high until completely smooth, about 30 seconds.
6. Chill in the refrigerator and serve cold with an assortment of cut raw vegetables for dipping into hummus.
7. Bon appétit!

Nutrition

- Calories: 203
- Fat: 11g
- Carbohydrate: 20g
- Protein: 4g

Pressure Cooker Nomato Sauce

Servings: 6 cups

Prep Time: 10 mins

Cook Time: 25 mins

Total Time: 35 mins

Ingredients

- 2 tbsp olive oil
- 1 large onion, diced
- 5 ribs celery, diced
- 8 carrots, diced
- 8 cloves of garlic, diced
- 1 small butternut squash, peeled and cubed
- 4 beets, peeled and diced
- 1/4 cup fresh lemon juice
- 1 cup broth
- 2 bay leaves
- 1 small bunch fresh basil, roughly chopped
- 1/2 tsp sea salt

Instructions

1. Add olive oil to Instant Pot and press the sauté button.
2. Add onion, celery, and carrots and cook for 4-5 minutes, stirring occasionally.
3. Add garlic and sauté for an additional 1-2 minutes or until the vegetables begin to soften.
4. Hit the cancel button to stop the sauté mode.
5. Add remaining ingredients and stir until evenly combined.
6. Put lid on Instant Pot and flip vent to sealing.
7. Cook on manual for 12 minutes and quick release the pressure.
8. Remove bay leaves and use an immersion blender to puree into a sauce.
9. Serve warm. Keep refrigerated for up to 5 days or freeze for another day.

Nutrition

- Calories: 65.4
- Fat: 2.4g
- Carbohydrate: 9.7g
- Protein: 1.4g

Silky Sweet Potato Puree [AIP-Friendly/Whole30]

Servings: 6

Prep Time: 5 minutes

Cook Time: 15 minutes

Total Time: 20 minutes

Ingredients

- 2 lbs white sweet potatoes, peeled and chopped into 1-inch cubes
- 1 1/2 cups beef or pork bone broth
- 1/2 tsp sea salt

Instructions

1. Place sweet potatoes and bone broth in your Instant Pot.
2. Set timer to 10 minutes and let pressure cook until potatoes easily break apart with a fork.
3. Alternatively, you can steam the sweet potatoes by placing them in a steamer basket fitted in a pot with the bone broth.
4. Bring to a low boil, cover with a lid, and let the sweet potatoes, steam cook, for 15 minutes.
5. Pour sweet potatoes, broth, and sea salt into Vitamix, Blendtec, or food processor.
6. Blend on medium speed for at least 30 seconds until a very silky puree has formed.
7. Serve with your favorite prepared meat or seafood dish!

Nutrition

- Calories: 130
- Fat: 0g
- Carbohydrate: 30g
- Protein: 3g

Savoy Cabbage with Cream Sauce (Wirsing it Sahnesoße)

Servings: 4 - 6

Prep Time: 10 mins

Cook Time: 10 mins

Total Time: 20 mins

Ingredients

- 1 cup bacon/lardons, diced
- 1 onion, chopped
- 2 cups bone broth
- 1 medium head Savoy cabbage, chopped finely (about 2lb)
- ¼ tsp mace (Use nutmeg if you have reintroduced this successfully while on the AIP)
- ½ can or 200ml coconut milk (scant 1 cup)
- 1 bay leaf
- Sea salt, to taste
- 2 tbsp parsley flakes

Instructions

1. Prepare a parchment round by tracing around the inner pot on a piece of parchment paper and then cutting it out.
2. Press Sauté and allow the inner pot to heat up.
3. Once 'Hot' is displayed, fry the bacon and onions in the inner pot until the bacon is crisp and the onions are lightly browned and translucent.
4. Add in the bone broth and scrape the bottom of the pot to remove any stuck browned bits.
5. Stir in the cabbage and bay leaf.
6. Cover with the parchment round and shut the lid, setting the sealing valve to 'sealing'.
7. Select 'Manual' and adjust the cooking time to 4 minutes.
8. Once the Instant Pot beeps at the end of the cooking cycle, press 'Keep warm/ cancel' and release the pressure before uncovering and removing the parchment round.
9. Press Sauté, bring to a boil and add in the mace or nutmeg and coconut milk.
10. Simmer for 5 minutes, then turn off the Instant Pot and stir in the parsley flakes before serving.

Nutrition

- Calories: 27
- Fat: 0.1g
- Carbohydrate: 6.1g
- Protein: 2g

Instant Pot Pressure-Steamed Artichokes

Servings: 1-2 (Each artichoke as an appetizer)

Prep Time: 5 mins

Cook Time: 20 mins

Total Time: 25 mins

Ingredients

- Whole artichokes (no more than you can fit upright in a single layer)
- 1 lemon wedge
- 1 cup water

Instructions

1. Rinse the artichokes with water and remove any damaged outer leaves.
2. Using a sharp knife, carefully trim off the stem and top third of each artichoke.
3. Rub the cut top with a lemon wedge to prevent browning.
4. Set the steam rack or a steamer basket into the Instant Pot's cooking insert, place the artichokes on top, and pour in a cup of water.
5. Close the lid and ensure that the valve is set to sealed position.
6. Select "Manual" mode, leave the setting on High Pressure, and adjust the time based on the size of your artichokes: 5 minutes for small, 10 minutes for medium, 15 minutes for large.
7. When the cooking time is up, wait 10 minutes before opening the valve to release any remaining pressure.
8. Use tongs to remove the artichokes from the cooker and serve warm with the dipping sauce of your choice.

Nutrition

- Calories: 59.3
- Fat: 2.5g
- Carbohydrate: 8.8g
- Protein: 2.5g

Quick Onion Soup {AIP}

Servings: 6

Prep Time: 30 minutes

Cook Time: 35 minutes

Total Time: 1 hour 5 minutes

Ingredients

- 2 tbsp / 30 ml avocado oil, coconut oil or good quality lard
- 8 cups / 960 g yellow onions
- 1 tbsp / 15 ml balsamic vinegar
- 6 cups / 1.4 L pork stock
- 1 tsp / 5g real salt
- 2 bay leaves
- 2 large sprigs of fresh thyme

Instructions

1. Cut the onions in half through the root, peel them and slice them into thin half-moons. Set the Instant Pot to Sauté and add the oil.
2. Once the oil is hot, add the onions.
3. Cook the onions until they have reduced down and become translucent, stirring occasionally to prevent sticking, about 15 minutes.
4. Add the balsamic vinegar and scrape up any food from the bottom of the Instant Pot, then add the stock, salt, bay leaves and thyme.
5. Turn off the Instant Pot and close the lid of the Instant Pot, making sure to check that the float is free and the vent isn't blocked and that the lid is set in the "Sealing" position.
6. Set the Instant Pot to "High Pressure" and cook the soup for 10 minutes once it has come up to pressure.
7. Allow the pressure to release using the "natural release" – don't open the vent or hot liquid may gush out of the vent along with the steam.
8. Discard the bay leaves and thyme stems, then blend the soup together either using an immersion blender directly in the pot or by transferring the soup carefully to a blender

Nutrition

- Calories: 290
- Fat: 9.6g
- Carbohydrate: 33.4g
- Protein: 16.8g

AIP Paleo Butternut Squash Soup

Servings: 6

Prep Time: 20 minutes

Cook Time: 25 minutes

Total Time: 45 minutes

Ingredients

- 1 whole organic butternut squash, peeled and chopped
- 1 whole organic onion or half of a huge onion, chopped
- 1 quart organic chicken stock (preferably your own bone broth)
- 1 tsp. organic ground cinnamon
- 1/2 tsp. organic ground nutmeg (optional)
- 1 tbsp. salt
- 2 tbsp organic avocado oil or coconut oil
- Optional 1/8 cup chopped pecans or other nuts that you tolerate for garnish

Instructions

1. Turn Instant Pot to Sauté.
2. Saute chopped onion in avocado oil.
3. When translucent add in cinnamon, nutmeg, and salt.
4. Add chopped butternut squash to pot and pour in broth.
5. Turn off Instant Pot.
6. Turn back on to Manual for 2 minutes.
7. Quick-release the pressure.
8. Pour into Vitamix and puree so it fills the Vitamix almost completely to the top.
9. Garnish with a sprinkle of cinnamon and chopped pecans (or nut of choice).

Nutrition

- Calories: 80
- Fat: 1.1g
- Carbohydrate: 17.9g
- Protein: 2.5g

Pressure Cooker Applesauce

Servings: 1 quart

Prep Time: 15 minutes

Cook Time: 20 minutes

Total Time: 35 minutes

Ingredients

- 12 medium apples, cored and diced (peeled if preferred)
- Scant ½ cup apple juice/non-alcoholic cider or water

Instructions

1. Place the apples in the inner pot of the Instant Pot.
2. Add in the apple juice or water.
3. Cut a circle of parchment paper large enough to fit just nicely within the inner pot and place it over the apples.
4. Cover the lid and set the pressure valve to 'Sealing'.
5. Press 'Manual' setting and adjust cooking time to 10 minutes.
6. Once cooking time is over, release the pressure naturally.
7. Uncover and discard the parchment paper circle.
8. Blend until smooth with a hand-held immersion blender or use a food mill.

Nutrition

- Calories: 101
- Fat: 0g
- Carbohydrate: 26g
- Protein: 0g

Chapter 9: Meat-Based (Main Dish) Recipes

Instant Pot Lemon Garlic Chicken

Servings: 8

Prep Time: 5 minutes

Cook Time: 15 minutes

Total Time: 20 minutes

Ingredients

- 1–2 pounds chicken breasts or thighs
- 1 teaspoon of sea salt
- 1 onion, diced
- 1 tablespoon avocado oil, lard, or ghee
- 5 garlic cloves, minced
- 1/2 cup organic chicken broth or homemade
- 1 teaspoon dried parsley
- 1/4 teaspoon paprika (omit for AIP)
- 1/4 cup white cooking wine (omit for AIP)
- 1 large lemon juiced (or more to taste)
- 3–4 teaspoons (or more) arrowroot flour

Instructions

1. Turn your Instant Pot onto the Sauté feature and place in the diced onion and cooking fat.
2. Cook the onions for 5-10 minutes or until softened. You can also choose to cook until they start to brown.
3. Add in the remaining ingredients except for the arrowroot flour and secure the lid on your Instant Pot.
4. Select the "Poultry" setting and make sure your steam valve is closed (12-15 minutes on Manual if you do not have a Poultry setting).
5. Allow cook time to complete, release steam valve to vent and then carefully remove the lid.
6. At this point, you may thicken your sauce by making a slurry. To do this remove about 1/4 cup sauce from the pot, add in the arrowroot flour, and then reintroduce the slurry into the remaining liquid.
7. Stir and serve right away. This also reheats well as leftovers.

Nutrition

- Calories: 141
- Fat: 1.5g
- Carbohydrate: 3g
- Protein: 27.4g

Collada Chicken

Servings: 4

Prep Time: 15 mins

Cook Time: 15 mins

Total Time: 30 mins

Ingredients

- 2 pounds organic chicken thighs, cut into 1" chunks
- 1 cup fresh or frozen pineapple chunks
- 1/2 cup full fat coconut cream
- 1 teaspoon cinnamon
- 1/8 teaspoon salt
- 2 tablespoons coconut aminos
- 1/2 cup chopped green onion (garnish)

Instructions

1. Place all ingredients, except green onions, into Instant Pot. Close lid.
2. Press the Poultry button.
3. The pot will automatically set itself for 15 minutes, high pressure. Allow cooking.
4. Once cooking has stopped, turn off Instant Pot.
5. Let pressure release naturally for 10 minutes.
6. Carefully open the lid and remove from pot. Stir.
7. If you'd like to thicken the sauce a bit, simply stir in a teaspoon of arrowroot starch mixed with a tablespoon of water.
8. Then, press the Saute button. Cook until sauce thickens to your liking. Turn off Instant Pot.
9. Serve with green onion garnish.

Instant Pot Shredded Chicken

Servings: 4

Prep Time: 5 minutes

Cook Time: 20 minutes

Total Time: 25 minutes

Ingredients

- 4 pounds chicken breast
- ½ cup water or chicken broth
- 1 teaspoon salt
- ½ teaspoon black pepper

Instructions

1. Add all of the ingredients to the Instant Pot.
2. Secure the lid, close the pressure valve and cook for 20 minutes at high pressure.
3. Quick-release pressure.
4. Shred the chicken with two forks.
5. Store the chicken in an air-tight container with the liquid, to help keep the meat moist.

Nutrition

- Calories: 150
- Fat: 6g
- Carbohydrate: 16g
- Protein: 9g

Instant Pot Artichokes with Lemon Tarragon Dipping Sauce

Servings: 4

Prep Time: 10 mins

Cook Time: 20 mins

Total Time: 30 mins

Ingredients

- 4 artichokes, 5 to 6 ounces each
- 2 small lemons
- 2 cups poultry bone broth
- 1 tbsp finely chopped tarragon leaves
- 1 stalk celery
- 1/2 cup extra-virgin olive oil
- 1/4 tsp sea salt

Instructions

1. Trim the stems of the artichokes so that they are one inch in length. Cut off one inch of the "petals" from the opposite end of the artichokes. Discard the stems and petal tips.
2. Zest the lemons and set aside. Cut four thin slices (about 1/4-inch) from the middle of one zested lemon, removing any seeds.
3. Place the lemon slices in the Instant Pot and top each lemon slice with a trimmed artichoke, stem-side up. Pour in the broth around the artichokes.
4. Close and lock the lid. Press MANUAL for high pressure. Set cooking time to 20 minutes. Once the time is up, quickly release the pressure.
5. While the artichokes are cooking, make the dipping sauce. Finely chop fresh tarragon leaves. Trim both ends of one stalk of celery and chop into small pieces.
6. Peel the remaining lemon and cut the white pith away with a paring knife. Coarsely chop the fruit. Throw away the seeds.
7. Place the lemon zest, lemon fruit, tarragon, chopped celery, olive oil, and salt in a blender or food processor and blend until thick and creamy.
8. Serve the artichokes with the dipping sauce. Feel free to drink the broth remaining in the Instant Pot.

Nutrition

- Calories: 59.3
- Fat: 2.5g
- Carbohydrate: 8.8g
- Protein: 2.5g

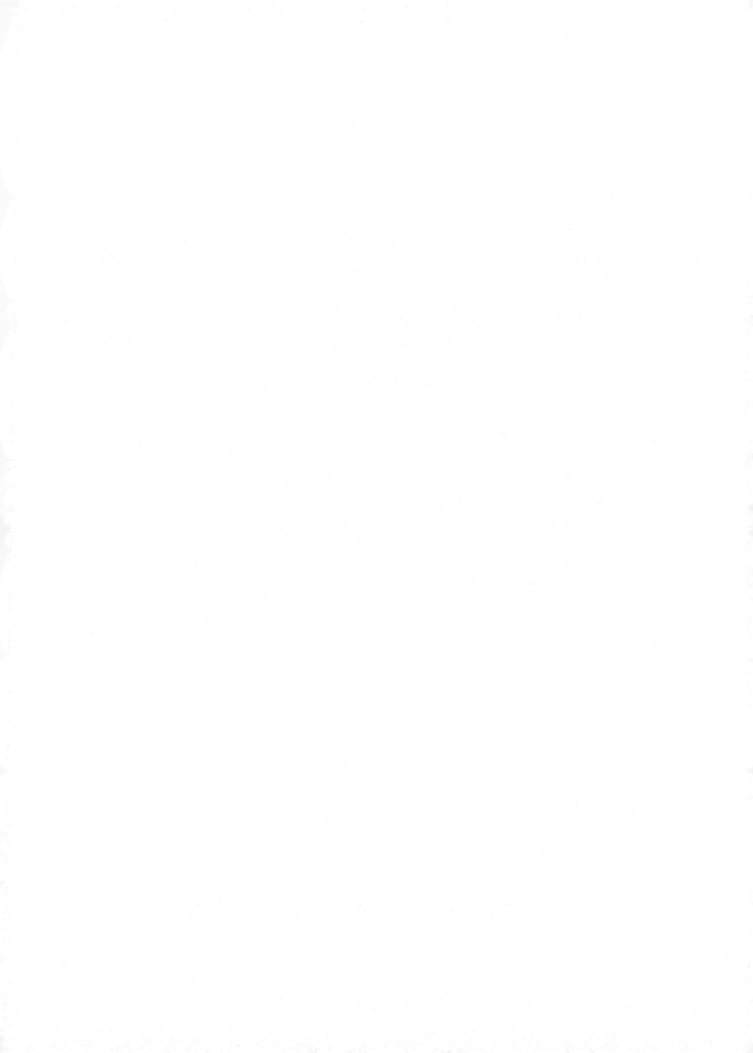

AIP Pressure Cooker Onion Soup

Servings: 2

Prep Time: 10 mins

Cook Time: 10 mins

Total Time: 20 mins

Ingredients

- 2 tablespoons (30 ml) of olive oil
- 2 large onions (220 g), peeled and sliced
- 2 garlic cloves (6 g), peeled
- 3 cups (720 ml) of best-quality fresh beef broth (warm)
- 2 teaspoons (10 ml) of coconut aminos
- Salt fresh thyme, to garnish

Instructions

1. Heat the olive oil in a pressure cooker on the stovetop and add the sliced onions. Cook over moderately high heat until they start to darken and caramelize.
2. Add the garlic and continue to cook the mixture until very dark and jammy. Do not allow the mixture to burn, but you do want to get a lot of color on the onions.
3. Pour in the warm beef broth and bring to a simmer. Secure the lid of the pressure cooker and cook under full pressure for 30 minutes.
4. Allow the pressure cooker to decompress before safely removing the lid.
5. Season the soup with a little coconut aminos and salt. Divide between two bowls and garnish with fresh thyme leaves.

Nutrition

- Calories: 201
- Fat: 16 g
- Carbohydrates: 11 g
- Protein: 1 g

Instant Pot Indian Curry Lamb Spare Ribs

Servings: 4

Prep Time: 10 mins

Marinating time: 4 hrs

Cook Time: 35 mins

Total Time: 4 hrs 45 mins

Ingredients

For the lamb spare ribs:

- 2½ pounds lamb spare ribs
- 2 teaspoons Diamond Crystal kosher salt
- 1 tablespoon Indian curry powder

For the sauce:

- 1 tablespoon coconut oil or ghee
- 1 large yellow onion, coarsely chopped
- ½ pound tomatoes, coarsely chopped
- 5 medium garlic cloves, minced
- 1 tablespoon Indian curry powder
- 1 tablespoon Diamond Crystal kosher salt
- 2 tablespoons freshly squeezed lemon juice
- 1¼ cup chopped cilantro, divided
- 4 scallions, thinly sliced

Instructions

1. Toss the lamb spare ribs with 2 teaspoons kosher salt and 1 tablespoon Indian curry powder. Cover and refrigerate for a minimum of four hours and up to a day.
2. When you're ready to cook off the ribs, melt the coconut oil or ghee on the Sauté function of your Instant Pot. Brown the spare ribs in two batches and remove them to a plate when they're done.
3. While the ribs are sizzling, grab the onion and tomatoes and toss them in a blender. Blitz until smooth.
4. After the lamb is seared, add minced garlic to the cooking fat in the empty Instant Pot insert. Stir the garlic until fragrant (30 seconds) before adding the tomato and onion puree.
5. Mix in 1 tablespoon Indian curry powder, 1 tablespoon kosher salt, 1 cup chopped cilantro, and lemon juice. Stir in the seared lamb spare ribs.
6. Lock on the pressure cooker lid and cook for 20 minutes under high pressure. When the ribs are done cooking, wait for the pressure to release naturally (10-15 minutes).

7. Scoop the grease off the top and discard. Taste and adjust for seasoning and stir in scallions and remaining ¼ cup chopped cilantro. Serve!

Nutrition

- Calories: 524
- Carbohydrates: 9g
- Protein: 58g
- Fat: 27g

Pressure Cooker Lamb Shanks

Servings: 4

Prep Time: 15 mins

Cook Time: 45 mins

Total Time: 1 hr

Ingredients

- 3 pounds lamb shanks
- Diamond Crystal kosher salt
- 2 tablespoons ghee, divided
- 2 medium carrots, roughly chopped
- 2 celery stalks, roughly chopped
- 1 large onion, roughly chopped
- 1 tablespoon tomato paste
- 3 garlic cloves, smashed and peeled
- 1 pound ripe roma tomatoes or 1 (14-ounce) can diced tomatoes, drained
- 1 cup bone broth
- 1 teaspoon Red Boat fish sauce
- 1 tablespoon aged balsamic vinegar
- 1/4 cup minced Italian parsley (optional)

Instructions

1. Grab the shanks and season them with salt and pepper to taste.
2. Melt a tablespoon of ghee over high heat in a 6-quart pressure cooker. Sear the lamb shanks until browned on all sides (8-10 minutes).
3. While the lamb is browning, chop up your carrots, celery, onion, and tomatoes.
4. Remove the lamb shanks from the pot and plop them on a platter.
5. Lower the heat to medium and add the remaining tablespoon of ghee to the pressure cooker.
6. Add the carrots, celery, and onion to the pot, and season with salt and pepper.
7. Once the vegetables have turned translucent, add tomato paste and garlic cloves and stir for one minute.
8. Add the shanks back into the pot along with the tomatoes and pour in the bone broth, fish sauce, and balsamic vinegar.
9. Before locking on the lid, grind on some fresh pepper.
10. Lock on the lid. With the lid tightly sealed, bring the contents of the pot up to high pressure over high heat.
11. Once high pressure is reached, turn down the heat to the minimum level needed to maintain high pressure for 45 minutes. Usually, the "low" or "simmer" settings should work.
12. When the braised shanks are finished cooking, let the pressure drop naturally.

13. Plate the shanks and adjust the sauce for seasoning. Ladle the sauce on the shanks.
14. Mince the Italian parsley and sprinkle it on top of the braised meat.

Nutrition

- Calories: 711
- Carbohydrates: 12g
- Protein: 63g
- Fat: 44g

Lamb Shanks with Ginger and Figs (Pressure Cooker, AIP)

Serves: 4

Prep time: 20 mins

Cook time: 90 mins

Total time: 1 hr 50 mins

Ingredients

- 2 tablespoons coconut oil
- 4 12-ounce lamb shanks
- 1 large onion, sliced thinly pole-to-pole
- 2 tablespoons minced fresh ginger
- 2 tablespoons coconut aminos
- 2 tablespoons apple cider vinegar
- 2 teaspoons fish sauce
- 2-3 cloves garlic, finely minced
- 1½ cups bone broth
- 10 dried figs, stems cut off and halved lengthwise

Instructions

1. Turn Instant Pot on and press the "Saute" button (or set a 6-quart stovetop pressure cooker over medium heat). When hot, add 1 tablespoon coconut oil.
2. Place two of the lamb shanks in the pot and brown on all sides, turning occasionally. Transfer to a plate or bowl. Repeat with remaining tablespoon coconut oil and lamb shanks.
3. Add onion and ginger to empty pot and cook, stirring often, until softened (about 3 minutes).
4. Stir in the coconut aminos, vinegar, fish sauce, and garlic. Stir in the broth and figs, scraping up any browned bits. Return the shanks and any accumulated juices to the pressure cooker. Make sure the meaty portion of each shank is at least partially submerged in the liquid. Lock lid in place.
5. If using Instant Pot or other electric pressure cookers, set the machine to cook at high pressure for 1 hour. OR If using a stovetop pressure cooker, raise heat to high and bring the pot to high pressure, then reduce the heat as much as possible while maintaining the pressure and cook for 40 minutes.
6. If using Instant Pot, turn off the machine; do not allow it to go into keep-warm setting, and let its pressure return to normal naturally for 20-30 minutes. OR If using a stovetop pressure cooker, remove the pot from heat and allow its pressure to fall to normal naturally for about 20 minutes.
7. Unlock and open the cooker. Transfer the shanks to a serving platter. Skim the surface fat from the sauce in the cooker and discard. Ladle the sauce over the shanks.

8. Serve with white rice or cauli-rice.

Nutrition

- Calories: 171
- Fat: 11.1g
- Carbohydrate: 0g
- Protein: 17.9g

Instant Pot Kalua Pig

Servings: 8

Prep Time: 10 mins

Cook Time: 1 hr 50 mins

Total Time: 2 hrs

Ingredients

- 3 bacon slices
- 5 pounds bone-in pork shoulder roast
- 1½ tablespoons Red Alaea Hawaiian Coarse Sea Salt or ~1 tablespoon Red Alaea Hawaiian fine sea salt
- 5 peeled garlic cloves - optional
- 1 cup water
- 1 cabbage cored, and cut into 6 wedges

Instructions

1. Drape three pieces of bacon on the bottom of your Instant Pot. Press the "Sauté" button and in about a minute, your bacon will start sizzling. (If you're using a stovetop pressure cooker instead, line it with three pieces of bacon, crank the burner to medium, and start frying your bacon.)
2. Slice the pork roast into three equal pieces. If you've got some garlic on hand, use it! With a sharp paring knife, stab a few slits in each piece of pork, and tuck in the garlic cloves.
3. Carefully measure out the amount of salt you use. For this recipe, follow Judy Rodger's rule of thumb: use ¾ teaspoon of medium-coarse salt for every 1 pound of meat. (Using fine salt? Use about half that amount.)
4. Sprinkle the salt evenly over the pork. As you're seasoning the pig, you'll hear the bacon sputtering in the pressure cooker. Don't forget to flip the slices, and turn off the heat when the bacon is browned on both sides.
5. Place the salted pork on top of the bacon, keeping the meat in a single layer.
6. Pour in the water. Check your pressure cooker manual to see what the minimum amount of liquid is for your particular model, and adjust accordingly. (After some digging and experimenting, I discovered that 1 cup of water is perfect for this recipe in my Instant Pot.)
7. Cover and lock the lid.
8. If you're using an Instant Pot, select the "Manual" button and press the "+" button until you hit 90 minutes under high pressure. Once the pot is programmed, walk away.
9. If you're using a stove-top pressure cooker, cook on high heat until high pressure is reached. Then, reduce the heat to low to maintain high pressure for about 75 minutes.
10. When the stew is finished cooking, the Instant Pot will switch automatically to its "Keep Warm" mode. If you're at home, press the "Keep Warm/Cancel" button to turn off the cooker and let the pressure come down naturally more quickly.

11. If you're using a stove-top pressure cooker, remove the pot from the heat. In either case, let the pressure release naturally (which will take about 15 minutes).
12. Once the cooker is depressurized, check that the pork is fork-tender. If the meat's not yet fall-apart tender, you can always cook the pork under pressure for another 5-10 minutes to get the right texture.
13. Transfer the cooked pork to a large bowl, and taste the cooking liquid remaining in the pot. Adjust the seasoning with water or salt if needed.
14. Chop the cabbage head into six wedges and add them to the cooking liquid. Replace the lid and cook the cabbage under high pressure for 1-5 minutes (depending on the size of the wedges and how tender you like the cabbage). When the cabbage is done cooking, activate the quick-release valve to release the pressure.
15. While the cabbage is cooking, shred the pork. Once the cabbage is cooked, pile it on the pork and serve.

Nutrition

- Calories: 321
- Carbohydrates: 8g
- Protein: 47g
- Fat: 10g

Red-cooked Pork (Hong Shao Rou) - Paleo/ AIP

Servings: 4

Prep Time: 5 minutes

Cook Time: 2 hours

Total Time: 2 hours 5 minutes

Ingredients

- 2lb/ 900g fatty pork belly, cut into 1.5" or 3.8cm cubes
- 2 tbsp maple syrup
- 3 tbsp sherry
- 1 tbsp blackstrap molasses
- 2 tbsp coconut aminos
- 1 tsp sea salt
- Cup water or bone broth
- 1 1"/ 2.5cm length fresh ginger, peeled and smashed
- A few sprigs of coriander/ cilantro leaves, to garnish

Instructions

1. Fill a pot with enough water to cover the pork cubes and bring to boil over high heat.
2. Add the pork cubes and boil for 3 minutes, then drain and rinse off any scum or impurities.
3. Set aside the pork cubes in a colander to drain.
4. Heat the maple syrup in the inner pot of the Instant Pot on 'Sauté' setting.
5. Add the pork cubes to the heated maple syrup and brown the pork for approximately 10 minutes (use a splatter guard).
6. Add the rest of the ingredients to the pot.
7. Bring to a boil, then press cancel/ keep warm.
8. Seal the lid, and valve, then select 'manual' setting and adjust the cooking time to 25 minutes.
9. Allow the pressure to release naturally.
10. Open the lid and select 'Sauté' setting.
11. Bring the contents to a simmer until the sauce is sufficiently reduced and thickened to coat the pork cubes (or to your liking).
12. Serve with coriander/ cilantro leaves as a garnish.

Nutrition

- Calories: 295
- Fat: 20g
- Carbohydrate: 7.5g
- Protein: 17g

90-Minute Kalua Pork

Yield: 8 - 10

Prep Time: 5 mins

Cook Time: 90 mins

Total Time: 95 mins

Ingredients

- 1 4-5 pound pork shoulder (I prefer bone-in, but boneless works too)
- 1 teaspoon salt (Hawaiian or sea salt)
- 1/2 cup diced pineapple, (fresh or canned)
- 1 teaspoon fish sauce (I love Red Boat!)
- 1 tablespoon liquid smoke
- 1/2 cup water

Instructions

1. Season the pork with salt and add to the insert of your Instant Pot along with the pineapple, fish sauce, liquid smoke, and water. Lock on the lid and turn the valve to sealing.
2. Cook at high pressure for 90 minutes.
3. After 90 minutes, allow the steam to release naturally for 10-15 minutes, then turn the valve to venting.
4. Remove the pork from the Instant Pot and carefully pour out the juices into a jar. Pull the meat apart with two forks, removing any excess fat.
5. Once the fat rises to the top of the jar, remove it with a small ladle and discard it. Add some of the juices back to the pork, as desired.

Nutrition

- Calories: 269.5
- Fat: 20.4g
- Carbohydrate: 0g
- Protein: 9.9g

Paleo Lechon Asado (AIP / Instant Pot)

Servings: 6

Prep Time: 2 hours 10 minutes

Cook Time: 2 hours

Total Time: 4 hours 10 minutes

Ingredients

- 4-6 lb pork roast (Boston butt works well)
- 1 to 1.5 cups mojo criollo marinade (without oil)
- 1 onion thinly sliced
- 2 tbsp lard or olive oil (for Instant Pot method)

Instructions

1. Make the mojo criollo marinade
2. Place roast in a large bag with an air-tight seal (like Ziploc) and pour in marinade and sliced onion. Let sit overnight in the fridge.
3. Cut the roast into 2-4 smaller pieces. Press "Saute" to preheat the cooker.
4. When it says "hot", add fat to the bottom of the pot and brown all sides of each piece of meat.
5. Turn the IP off when done.
6. Add roast, marinade, and onion.
7. Press "manual". Make sure "high pressure" is selected.
8. Use the + button to increase the time to 90 minutes for a 4 lb roast.
9. When the roast finishes, allow the pressure to release naturally.
10. The meat will be falling-apart tender.
11. Remove, shred with 2 forks, and mix with some of the liquid that cooked out to keep it nice and juicy and flavorful. Serve with lime wedges and enjoy!
12. Save the extra cooking juices for braising greens –YUM!

Nutrition

- Calories: 481
- Fat: 40g
- Carbohydrate: 3g
- Protein: 23g

AIP Pork Belly & Spiced Rice

Servings: 4

Prep Time: 15 mins

Cook Time: 15 mins

Total Time: 30 mins

Ingredients

- 1 pound pork belly, cooked and cubed
- 4 cups riced cauliflower
- 1/2 cup bone broth
- 1/2 red onion, sliced
- 1/2 cup cilantro, divided
- 2 green onions, sliced
- 1 tablespoon lime juice
- 3 cloves garlic, sliced
- 1 tablespoon animal fat
- 1 teaspoon turmeric
- 1 tablespoon oregano
- 1 tablespoon cumin (optional; leave out for elimination phase of AIP)
- 1/2 teaspoon salt

Instructions

1. Place all ingredients in the Instant Pot.
2. Place lid on Instant Pot.
3. Press the Manual button.
4. Set time to 15 minutes.
5. Once the dish is done cooking, turn off Instant Pot.
6. Allow pressure to release naturally for 10 minutes before opening lid.

Nutrition

- Calories: 1628
- Fat: 165g
- Carbohydrate: 2.66g
- Protein: 29g

Pressure Cooker Porcini and Tomato Beef Short Ribs

Servings: 6

Prep Time: 15 mins

Cook Time: 45 mins

Total Time: 1 hr

Ingredients

- 5 pounds beef short ribs cut into 3- to 4-inch segments
- Diamond Crystal kosher salt
- Freshly ground black pepper
- 1/2 ounce dried porcini mushrooms
- 1 cup water
- 1 tablespoon ghee or fat of choice
- 1 large onion, chopped 2 celery stalks, chopped
- 6 cloves of garlic, peeled and smashed
- 1 cup marinara sauce
- 1/2 cup bone broth
- 2 tablespoon balsamic vinegar, divided
- 1/4 cup minced Italian parsley

Instructions

1. Season the short ribs liberally with salt and pepper.
2. Take out your pressure cooker or Instant Pot, and melt the ghee or fat over medium-high heat.
3. Sear the ribs in batches until well browned and transfer them to a platter.
4. While the ribs are browning, chop up the veggies and toss the onions, carrots, and celery into the empty pot.
5. Lower the heat to medium, season with salt and pepper, and sauté the vegetables until softened.
6. Toss the dried porcini mushrooms into the pot along with the garlic. Stir the pot for one minute.
7. Add in the marinara sauce, broth, and 1 tablespoon of the balsamic vinegar.
8. Add the ribs back into the pot, mixing well.
9. Increase the heat to high and bring the stew to a boil. Cover the pressure cooker with the lid and let the contents come to high pressure.
10. Once the pot reaches high pressure, decrease the heat to low and maintain high pressure for 30 minutes. Then, take the pot off the heat and let the pressure come down naturally (10-15 minutes).
11. When the pressure is released, add the remaining tablespoon of vinegar, check for seasoning, and top with minced parsley.

Nutrition

- Calories: 536
- Carbohydrates: 8g
- Protein: 55g
- Fat: 31g

Instant Pot (Pressure Cooker) Mexican Beef

Servings: 6

Prep Time: 15 mins

Cook Time: 45 mins

Total Time: 1 hr

Ingredients

- 2½ pounds boneless beef short ribs beef brisket, or beef chuck roast cut into 1½- to 2-inch cubes
- 1 tablespoon chili powder
- 1½ teaspoons Diamond Crystal kosher salt
- 1 tablespoon ghee or fat of choice
- 1 medium onion, thinly sliced
- 1 tablespoon tomato paste
- 6 garlic cloves, peeled and smashed
- ½ cup roasted tomato salsa
- ½ cup Instant Pot bone broth
- ½ teaspoon Red Boat fish sauce
- freshly ground black pepper
- ½ cup minced cilantro optional
- 2 radishes, thinly sliced (optional)

Instructions

1. In a large bowl, combine cubed beef, chili powder, and salt.
2. Press the "Sauté" button on your Instant Pot and add the ghee to the cooking insert.
3. Once the fat's melted, add the onions and sauté until translucent.
4. Stir in the tomato paste and garlic, and cook for 30 seconds or until fragrant.
5. Toss in the seasoned beef, and pour in the salsa, stock, and fish sauce.
6. Cover and lock the lid, and press the "Keep Warm/Cancel" button on the Instant Pot.
7. Press the "Manual" or "Pressure Cook" button to switch to the pressure cooking mode.
8. Program your IP to cook for 35 minutes under high pressure. If your cubes are smaller than mine, you can press the "minus" button to decrease the cooking time.
9. Once the pot is programmed, walk away.
10. When it's finished cooking, serve and enjoy!

Nutrition

- Calories: 381kcal
- Carbohydrates: 6g
- Protein: 38g
- Fat: 22g

Instant Pot Carne Guisada

Servings: 6

Prep Time: 10 minutes

Cook Time: 6 hours

Total Time: 6 hours 10 minutes

Ingredients

- 2 tablespoons avocado oil or fat of choice
- 1 pound beef stew meat
- 1 onion, diced
- 1 tablespoon minced garlic
- 1 Serrano pepper, minced
- 1 bay leaf

Spices

- 1 teaspoon ground cumin
- 1 teaspoon chili powder
- 1 teaspoon paprika
- 1 teaspoon salt
- ½ teaspoon pepper
- ½ teaspoon chipotle powder
- ½ teaspoon oregano
- 1 cup beef broth or chicken stock
- ½ cup tomato sauce
- 1 tablespoon potato starch or thickener of choice (optional)

Instructions

1. Press the sauté button on the Instant Pot, add the oil and beef cubes to the pot.
2. Sear the meat on all sides.
3. Once the meat has browned, add the onion, garlic, serrano pepper, bay leaf, and spices.
4. Stir-fry for 2-3 minutes.
5. Pour in the beef broth and tomato sauce.
6. Secure the lid, close the valve and cook for 35 minutes at high pressure.
7. Naturally release pressure.
8. Serve over cauli-rice, or in a tortilla!

Nutrition

- Calories: 217
- Fat: 6g

- Carbohydrate: 6g
- Protein: 31g

Instant Pot (Pressure Cooker) Mocha-Rubbed Pot Roast

Servings: 4

Prep Time: 10 mins

Cook Time: 50 mins

Total Time: 1 hr 10 mins

Ingredients

For the mocha rub:

- 2 tablespoons finely ground coffee (you can substitute decaf)
- 2 tablespoons smoked paprika
- 1 tablespoon freshly ground black pepper
- 1 tablespoon cocoa powder
- 1 teaspoon Aleppo pepper (you can substitute red pepper flakes)
- 1 teaspoon chili powder
- 1 teaspoon ground ginger
- 1 teaspoon of sea salt

For the roast:

- 2 pounds beef chuck roast cut into 1½- to 2-inch cubes
- 1 cup brewed coffee you can substitute decaf or broth
- 1 cup beef broth or bone broth
- 1 small onion, chopped
- 6 dried figs, chopped
- 3 tablespoons balsamic vinegar
- Kosher salt
- Freshly ground black pepper

Instructions

- Mix the ingredients for the mocha rub in a small bowl. You won't need all of the rubs, so save the extra in a tightly sealed container.
- Brew a cup of coffee. When I'm making just one cup, I turn to my Aeropress—not only because it makes a mean cuppa coffee, but also because it tickles me to know that the Aeropress was invented by the same dude who made Aerobie flying rings.
- Place the beef cubes in a large bowl and add three to four tablespoons of the mocha rub.
- Toss well until the beef is evenly coated.
- Combine the brewed coffee, broth, onion, figs, and balsamic vinegar in a high-powered blender. Blitz until liquefied.

- Transfer the seasoned beef to your pressure cooker and pour the sauce on top.
- Cover and lock the lid of your pressure cooker.
- If you're using an Instant Pot, turn it on and press the "Meat/Stew" button to switch it to the pressure cooking mode. And if your cubes are smaller than mine, you can press the "minus" button to decrease the cooking time from the preset 35-minute cooking time. Once the pot is programmed, walk away. (Or, if you're like me, sit down and eat dinner.)
- When the stew is finished cooking, the Instant Pot will switch automatically to a "Keep Warm" mode. At this point, turn it off and let the pressure release naturally (about 15 minutes).
- (Using a stove-top pressure cooker? You won't have all those buttons to press; instead, just cook on high heat until high pressure is reached. Then, reduce the heat to low to maintain high pressure for about 30 minutes. Remove the pot from the heat, and let the pressure release naturally.)
- Pop open the lid. The meat should be fork-tender. If it's not, cook it under high pressure for 5 more minutes.
- Transfer the cooked beef to a serving platter.
- Shred the meat with two forks.
- If desired, heat the remaining sauce to a boil to reduce and thicken it. Adjust the seasoning with salt and pepper to taste.
- Ladle the sauce on the beef and dig in!

Nutrition

- Calories: 489
- Carbohydrates: 17g
- Protein: 48g
- Fat: 27g

Pressure Cooker Pot Roast & Gravy

Servings: 4-6

Prep time: 5 mins

Cook time: 60 mins

Ingredients

- 4 pounds chuck roast, cut into 4 pieces
- a good pinch of salt
- freshly ground black pepper
- 1 1/2 cups beef broth
- 2 tablespoons balsamic vinegar
- 2 teaspoons fish sauce (optional, add more salt if omitting)
- 1 three-inch sprig rosemary
- 4 three-inch sprigs thyme
- 2 parsnips, peeled
- 4 carrots, peeled or scrubbed
- 6 cloves garlic, peeled
- chopped parsley and/or chives for serving, optional

Instructions

1. Season the beef with salt and pepper and place it in the pressure cooker.
2. Place all of the remaining ingredients in the pressure cooker.
3. Lock on the lid and set it for 60 minutes on high pressure.
4. After the 60 minutes are up, allow the pressure to release naturally for 15 minutes.
5. Remove the meat to a plate, and the veggies to a blender
6. Discard the rosemary and thyme stems.
7. Pour the cooking liquid into a large jar or measuring cup.
8. Once the fat rises to the top (this will happen quickly), remove and discard it with a large spoon or small ladle.
9. Pour the remaining liquid into the blender with the veggies and blend until smooth.
10. Season to taste with salt and pepper.
11. Roughly shred the meat using two forks.
12. Serve with your favorite roasted or mashed potatoes, cauliflower mash, or any root veggie, mashed or roasted.

Nutrition

- Calories: 180
- Carbohydrates: 4g
- Protein: 23g
- Fat: 8g

Pressure Cooker Grass Fed Beef Back Ribs

Servings: 4

Prep Time: 2 hrs 15 mins

Cook Time: 45 mins

Total Time: 3 hrs

Ingredients

- 3.5-pound grass-fed beef back ribs 1 rack
- dry rub of choice (I used Penzeys Chili 9000)
- Diamond Crystal kosher salt
- 3/4 cup water
- 4-ounce unsweetened applesauce
- 2 tablespoons coconut aminos
- 1 teaspoon fish sauce

Instructions

1. Grab a rack of grass-fed beef back ribs and pat it dry with a paper towel. Then, sprinkle it liberally on both sides with the dry rub and kosher salt.
2. Wrap it up in foil to marinate for at least two hours and up to a day.
3. When you're ready to cook the ribs, preheat the broiler with the rack positioned 4-6 inches from the heating element.
4. Grab the rack from the fridge and cut it so it'll fit in your pressure cooker. If you've got a 6-quart pot, cut the rack into three even pieces.
5. Put the chopped up ribs on a wire rack in a foil-lined, rimmed baking sheet.
6. Broil the ribs for 1-2 minutes on each side to get a nice char. Keep the broiler on because you'll be broiling these meaty bones again at the end.
7. Add the water, applesauce, coconut aminos, and fish sauce to the pressure cooker. Stir to combine and add a rack to the pot.
8. Pile the ribs into the pressure cooker and lock on the lid.
9. Crank the heat to high and when the pot reaches high pressure, turn down the heat to maintain high pressure on the lowest setting possible.
10. Cook on high pressure for 20 minutes and let the pressure come down naturally or release it quickly.
11. Remove the ribs and place them back on a wire rack atop a foil-lined, rimmed baking sheet.
12. Simmer the cooking liquid until it is reduced to 2 cups (~5 minutes). Skim off the excess fat at the top if desired and adjust seasoning.
13. Baste the racks with the braising liquid and boil them for about a minute to get some crunchy bits.

Nutrition

- Calories: 860kcal
- Carbohydrates: 5g
- Protein: 50g
- Fat: 100g

Instant Pot Butter Chicken

Servings: 2-3lbs chicken

Prep Time: 15 min

Cook Time: 17 min (8 min active cooking, 9 min coming to pressure)

Total Time: 32 min

Ingredients

- 2–3 lbs (family pack) boneless skinless chicken thighs (cut into bite-sized pieces)
- 1 tbsp ghee
- 1 1/2 large onions (chopped)
- 2 1/2 – 3 1/3 tsp salt
- 2 tsp garlic powder or 2 tbsp fresh garlic (minced)
- 2 tsp ginger powder or 2 tbsp fresh ginger (grated)
- 2 heaped tsp turmeric
- 2 heaped tsp paprika
- 1 1/2 tsp cayenne powder
- 1 1/2 – 2 cups stewed or canned tomatoes and the liquid
- 370 ml tomato paste
- 2 400ml cans coconut milk (*NOT the coconut drink – see link* – Allow these to separate – DO NOT shake. Best if left in the fridge overnight)
- 2 heaped tsp garam masala
- 1/2 cup sliced almondS
- 1/2 cup cilantro

Instructions

1. Melt ghee.
2. Add 2 tsp salt and onions.
3. Cook until onions are soft and translucent
4. Add in garlic, ginger, turmeric, paprika, and cayenne.
5. Mix in and cook until fragrant.
6. Add canned tomatoes and the watery portion of coconut milk.
7. Mixing thoroughly with spices (getting all of the spices stuck to the bottom of the pan).
8. Add chicken and stir well.
9. Once cooked, use the quick release of pressure, stir in coconut cream, tomato paste, garam masala and most of the cilantro.
10. Add more salt if needed.
11. Top with sliced almonds and garnish with more cilantro.
12. Enjoy!

Nutrition

- Calories: 150
- Fat: 11g
- Carbohydrate: 13g
- Protein: 1g

Fall-Off-The-Bone Pressure Cooker Chicken AIP

Servings: 10

Prep Time: 10 mins

Cook Time: 35 mins

Total Time: 45 mins

Ingredients

- 1 whole – 4lb. organic chicken
- 1 tbsp. organic virgin coconut oil
- 1 tsp. paprika
- 1 1/2 cups Pacific organic bone broth (chicken)
- 1 tsp. dried thyme
- 1/4 tsp. freshly ground black pepper
- 2 tbsp. lemon juice
- 1/2 tsp. sea salt
- 6 cloves garlic, peeled

Instructions

1. In a small bowl, combine paprika, thyme, salt, and pepper.
2. Rub seasoning over outside of the bird.
3. Heat oil in the pressure cooker to shimmering.
4. Add chicken, breast side down, and cook 6-7 minutes.
5. Flip the chicken and add broth, lemon juice, and garlic cloves.
6. Lock pressure cooker lid and set for 25 minutes on high.
7. Let the pressure cooker release naturally.
8. Remove from the pressure cooker and let stand for 5 minutes before carving.

Nutrition

- Calories: 224
- Fat: 7g
- Carbohydrate: 1.1g
- Protein: 39g

Cherry Tomato Pressure Cooker Chicken Cacciatore

Serves: 4-6

Prep time: 5 mins

Cook time: 22 mins

Total time: 27 mins

Ingredients

- 1 teaspoon olive oil
- 3 pounds (1.5 kilos) bone-in chicken legs and thighs
- 1 pound (500g) cherry tomatoes
- 2 garlic cloves, crushed.
- ¼ teaspoon hot pepper flakes (or one fresh hot pepper, chopped)
- 1 teaspoon salt (use 2 teaspoons if your chicken has not been previously salt-brined)
- 1 teaspoon dried oregano
- ¼ cup (60ml) tart red table wine (such as Merlot)
- 1 cup water
- 1 sprig fresh basil leaves, torn
- ½ cup (70g) pitted green olives, rinsed

Instructions

1. In the heated pressure cooker, add the olive oil and brown the chicken thighs on all sides.
2. In the meantime, remove the stems from the cherry tomatoes and put them in a large Ziploc bag so they are in a single layer. Close the bag almost completely - leave a tiny hole at the end. Or loosely knot a common plastic bag.
3. With a meat pounder, or heavy pot, lightly crush all of the cherry tomatoes - the goal is to burst them open, not flatten them.
4. Set the chicken aside and pour the crushed cherry tomato mixture and all of its juice into the pressure cooker base.
5. Add the garlic, hot pepper, salt, oregano, wine, and water and mix well, scraping up the brown bits of chicken stuck to the bottom of the cooker.
6. Place the chicken back into the pressure cooker and mix to coat the chicken with the contents of the cooker. Then, "smooth" out the chicken pieces into an even layer.
7. Close and lock the lid of the pressure cooker.
8. For electric pressure cookers: Cook for 13-14 minutes at high pressure.
9. For stovetop pressure cookers: Turn the heat up to high and when the cooker indicates it has reached high pressure, lower to the heat to maintain it and begin counting 12 minutes pressure cooking time.
10. When time is up, open the cooker by releasing the pressure through the valve.

11. Stir the contents and let the cooker stand uncovered for about 5 minutes, stirring occasionally to reduce some of the cooking liquid using the pressure cooker's residual heat.
12. Using a slotted spoon, lift into a serving casserole and sprinkle with green olives and basil before serving.
13. Reserve the broth left in the base of the pressure cooker to use in place of stock in a risotto or rice recipe.

Nutrition

- Calories: 81.3
- Fat: 6.4g
- Carbohydrate: 6.6g
- Protein: 4.3g

Swedish Meatballs - AIP Instant Pot

Servings: 6-8

Prep Time: 15 mins

Cook Time: 20 mins

Total Time: 35 mins

Ingredients

- 1 pound ground beef
- 1 pound ground pork
- ¼ cup minced fresh parsley, divided
- 2 tablespoons dried minced onion
- 1 teaspoon dried sage
- ½ teaspoon ground mace
- ½ teaspoon of sea salt
- 2 cups sliced mushrooms - button or crimini
- 1 large onion, chopped
- ½ cup bone broth (or coconut milk or water)
- 3 tablespoons coconut aminos
- (optional non-AIP spices: a pinch of nutmeg, allspice, black pepper and/or crushed fennel seed)

Instructions

1. In a bowl mix together ground beef, pork, 3 tablespoons minced parsley, dried onion, sage, mace, and salt.
2. Once thoroughly mixed, form into meatballs about 1-inch in diameter.
3. Place mushrooms, onion, broth/coconut milk/water, and coconut aminos into the Instant Pot.
4. Add the meatballs. Close and lock the lid.
5. Press the meat/stew button and set the cooking time to 20 minutes.
6. Once the time is up, very carefully quick release the pressure.
7. Using a slotted spoon gently remove meatballs and transfer to a serving platter.
8. Using an immersion blender or a high-speed blender, purée the cooked mushrooms, onions, and broth into a nice creamy gravy.
9. If the gravy is too thick, add a little more bone broth/coconut milk/water until the right consistency is reached.
10. Pour gravy over meatballs and garnish with remaining tablespoon of minced parsley.
11. This dish makes a wonderful appetizer as is, or the main course when served over spaghetti squash, cauliflower rice, sautéed veggies or warmed zucchini noodles

Nutrition

- Calories: 190

- Fat: 14g
- Carbohydrate: 4g
- Protein: 11g

AIP Pressure Cooker Chicken Curry

Servings: 6

Prep Time: 5 mins

Cook Time: 25 mins

Total Time: 30 mins

Ingredients

- 6 chicken thighs (900 g)
- 1 tablespoon (15 ml) of coconut oil
- 1 tablespoon (6 g) of turmeric
- 2 teaspoons (4 g) of ginger powder
- 1 cup (240 ml) of coconut milk
- Chopped fresh cilantro, to garnish

Instructions

1. Season both sides of the chicken thighs with salt.
2. Melt the coconut oil in a pressure cooker and fry the chicken thighs, skin-side down, until golden brown and crispy.
3. Remove the chicken thighs with a slotted spoon and set aside skin-side up.
4. If desired, pour out any excess rendered fat from the pressure cooker.
5. Add turmeric, ginger powder, and coconut milk to the pressure cooker and use a whisk to combine.
6. Cook the curry sauce, whisking continually, for a minute or two until slightly thick.
7. Place the chicken thighs skin-side up in the pressure cooker and secure the lid.
8. Cook over moderate heat for 14 to 15 minutes t.
9. Let the pressure decompress naturally before safely removing the lid.
10. Remove the chicken thighs from the pressure cooker with a slotted spoon and set aside to keep warm. Over high heat, reduce the remaining coconut sauce, whisking frequently to prevent burning, until thick to your liking.
11. Season the sauce with additional salt, if desired.
12. Pour the sauce over the chicken thighs and garnish with the chopped fresh cilantro.
13. Serve the chicken thighs and sauce immediately.

Nutrition

- Calories: 293
- Fat: 24 g
- Carbohydrates: 2 g
- Protein: 17 g

Pressure Cooker Beef And Broccoli

Servings: 2

Prep Time: 5 mins

Cook Time: 15 mins

Total Time: 20 mins

Ingredients

- 1 tablespoon (15 ml) of olive oil
- 14 oz (400 g) of beef sirloin, cut into bite-size pieces
- 1 teaspoon (2 g) of ginger paste (or minced fresh ginger)
- 1 teaspoon (2 g) of garlic paste (or 1 minced garlic clove)
- 1/2 cup (120 ml) of beef broth
- 1 ½ tablespoon (23 ml) of coconut aminos
- 1/2 head (8 oz or 225 g) of broccoli, broken into small florets
- Salt, to taste
- Sliced green onion, to garnish

Instructions

- Add the olive oil to the pressure cooker.
- Add the beef to the pressure cooker and saute until browned.
- Add the ginger paste and garlic paste to the pressure cooker and saute for about 30 seconds.
- Add the beef broth, coconut aminos, and broccoli florets to the pressure cooker and stir to combine.
- Place the lid on the pressure cooker and secure it to close it.
- Set the pressure cooker to cook for 10 minutes.
- Allow the pressure to release naturally before carefully removing the lid.
- Use a slotted spoon to remove the beef and broccoli from the pressure cooker and set aside.
- Reduce the liquid in the pressure cooker by half to create the sauce.
- Season with salt, to taste.
- Divide the beef and broccoli between 2 plates and drizzle with equal amounts of sauce.
- Garnish each plate with the sliced green onions.

Nutrition

- Calories: 635
- Fat: 49 g
- Carbohydrates: 8 g
- Protein: 37 g

AIP Pressure Cooker Pot Roast

Servings: 4

Prep Time: 10 mins

Cook Time: 1 hr

Total Time: 1 hr 10 mins

Ingredients

- 2 tablespoons (30 ml) of olive oil
- 1.12 lbs or 18 oz (504 g) of beef roast
- 1 large onion (110 g), peeled and quartered
- 2 cloves (6 g) of garlic, peeled and sliced
- 2 large carrots (100 g), peeled and cut into chunks
- 1 large zucchini (120 g), cut into very large chunks
- 10 white button mushrooms (100 g)
- 10.6 oz (318 ml) of beef stock
- 2 bay leaves
- 2 sprigs thyme, leaves picked
- AIP gravy, to serve

Instructions

- Heat the oil in a pressure cooker and brown the beef roast on all sides.
- Add the onion, garlic, and carrot to the pan and cook until slightly caramelized.
- Add the zucchini, mushrooms, beef stock, and herbs.
- Secure the lid of the pressure cooker and cook for 40-45 minutes.
- Allow the pressure cooker to cool slightly and decompress before safely opening the lid.
- Remove the beef and the vegetables with a slotted spoon and place onto a serving platter.
- Allow to rest for 10 minutes before slicing and serving with AIP gravy.

Nutrition

- Calories: 432
- Fat: 34 g
- Carbohydrates: 7 g
- Protein: 23 g

Instant Pot Pineapple Chicken

Servings: 6

Prep time: 5 mins

Cook time: 25 mins

Total time: 30 mins

Ingredients

Dump & Cook:

- 2 lbs chicken thighs   (cut into 1-2 inch pieces)
- 1/3 cup low sodium soy sauce
- 2 tablespoons sesame oil
- 1 20 oz can pineapple chucks (do NOT drain)
- 1 tablespoon minced garlic
- 1 tablespoon ginger grated
- 1/2 cup brown sugar
- 1/3 cup hoisin sauce
- 1 teaspoon red pepper flakes (optional)

Cornstarch Slurry:

- 2 tablespoons pineapple juice
- 2 tablespoons cornstarch

Garnish:

- 4 green onions sliced
- Sesame seeds
- Slivered almonds

Instructions

1. Open the pineapple can, set aside 1/4 cup of juice - the rest will be added to the pressure cooker, so make sure you save this.
2. Add all the ingredients from the "Dump & Cook" section to the Instant Pot: chicken, soy sauce, sesame oil, garlic, ginger, hoisin sauce, red pepper flakes, brown sugar, and canned pineapple chunks with juice (except the 1/4 cup).
3. Stir well to combine all the ingredients.
4. Close lid, make sure the pressure cooker is sealed. Select the Poultry function and adjust the time to 5 minutes on High Pressure. Or just select Manual, and select 5 minutes on High Pressure.
5. Use a 10-minute Natural Release. Turn off the heat. Release the remaining pressure. Open the lid.

6. Select again the Sauté function, on LOW.
7. In a small bowl combine 2 tablespoons of cornstarch with 2 tablespoons of pineapple juice, and whisk until all combined with no lumps.
8. Add the mixture to the Instant Pot and gently stir to combine. Cook on Sauté function for a few more minutes, stirring gently, until the sauce thickens.
9. If you want the sauce even thicker, mix one more tablespoon of cornstarch with 1 tablespoon of juice and add it to the pressure cooker.
10. Let the chicken stand for 5-7 minutes; the sauce will thicken more.
11. Serve over rice and garnish with freshly chopped green onions, sesame seeds, and slivered almonds.

Nutrition

- Calories: 561
- Carbohydrates: 46
- Protein: 26
- Fat: 30

Pressure Cooker Italian Beef

Servings: 6-8

Prep Time: 5 mins

Cook Time: 2 hrs 5 mins

Total Time: 2 hrs 10 mins

Ingredients

- 3 lb grass-fed chuck roast
- 6 cloves garlic
- 2 tsp garlic powder
- 1 tsp onion powder
- 1/2 tsp ground ginger
- 1 tsp oregano
- 1 tsp basil
- 1 tsp marjoram
- 1 tsp Himalayan pink salt
- 1 cup beef broth
- 1/4 cup apple cider vinegar

Instructions

1. Cut slits into the roast and stuff with garlic cloves.
2. Whisk garlic powder, onion powder, ground ginger, oregano, basil, marjoram, and salt until well combined.
3. Rub seasoning blend on all sides of the roast and place in the Instant Pot.
4. Pour beef broth and apple cider vinegar into the pot.
5. Seal the lid and make sure the valve is closed.
6. Press Manual and set time to 90 minutes.
7. It should take approximately 15 minutes to come to pressure.
8. Allow to natural release (approximately 20 minutes).
9. Remove beef from pot and shred with two forks or caveman claws.
10. Add juice if desired.

Nutrition

- Calories: 140
- Fat: 7g
- Carbohydrate: 0g
- Protein: 18g

Low-Carb Pork Roast with Cauliflower Gravy

Servings: 4

Prep Time: 20 minutes

Cook Time: 2 hours

Total Time: 2 hours 20 minutes

Ingredients

- 2 to 3-pound pork roast - preferably a fatty cut
- 1 teaspoon sea salt
- 1/2 teaspoon black pepper
- 4 cups chopped cauliflower
- 1 medium onion
- 4 cloves garlic
- 2 ribs celery
- 8 ounces portabello mushrooms sliced
- 2 tablespoons organic coconut oil (unrefined) or ghee
- 2 cups water, filtered

Instructions

1. At the bottom of your pressure cooker, place cauliflower, onion, garlic, celery, and water.
2. Top with pork roast and season with sea salt & pepper.
3. Cook under pressure for 90 minutes if your roast is frozen, 60 minutes if completely thawed.
4. Quick depressurize following manufacturer's directions.
5. Carefully remove the pork roast from the pressure cooker and place it in an ovenproof dish.
6. Bake at 400 degrees while preparing the gravy; this helps to render the fat and crisp up the edges of the pork to be more like as if it had been slow roasted.
7. Transfer cooked vegetables and broth to your blender and blend until smooth, then set aside.
8. In your (dirty) pressure cooker (on the saute function) cook mushrooms in coconut oil until soft, roughly 3-5 minutes.
9. Add blended vegetables and continue to cook on the Sauté function until it is thickened as desired.
10. Serve mushroom gravy over shredded pork.

Nutrition

- Calories: 407
- Fat: 28.3g
- Carbohydrate: 12.5g
- Protein: 27.1g

Beef and Plantain Curry

Servings: 5-6

Prep Time: 10 minutes

Cook Time: 1 hour 40 minutes

Total Time: 1 hour 50 minutes

Ingredients

- 2 tsp coconut oil
- 1 tsp garlic powder
- 1 tsp ginger powder
- 1 tsp turmeric powder
- 1 tsp sea salt
- 2lbs bottom blade pot roast, cut into 1.5 – 2-inch cubes
- 2 small onions, peeled and thinly sliced
- 3 tsp coconut oil
- 1 cup coconut milk
- 4 kaffir lime leaves
- 1 stick cinnamon
- 1 very ripe plantain (mostly black), sliced lengthwise and cut into 1-inch chunks
- Sea salt, to taste
- 1 tbsp coriander leaves, chopped

Instructions

1. In a small bowl, combine garlic powder, ginger powder, turmeric, powder and sea salt with 2 tsp coconut oil.
2. Marinate beef with spice mixture for about 1 hour.
3. Using the 'Saute' function of the Instant Pot, cook the onions in 3tsp coconut oil until translucent.
4. Remove and set aside.
5. Working in batches, brown the marinated meat in the pressure cooker pot until seared on all sides.
6. Top up with extra oil if necessary. Set aside.
7. Pour the coconut milk into the pot, stirring gently to remove any browned bits of meat stuck to the bottom of the pot.
8. Add in the onions, browned meat, kaffir lime leaves, and cinnamon stick.
9. Cook for 35 minutes on the Manual setting.
10. Once the cooking time is completed, allow the cooker to cool naturally until the pressure is released.
11. Select the 'Saute' function and add in the plantain, stirring gently to mix.

12. Add sea salt to taste.
13. Let it simmer until the plantain is cooked and the gravy has thickened slightly. If the plantain is very ripe, it should not take more than 5 minutes.
14. Remove the cinnamon stick and kaffir lime leaves.
15. Sprinkle with chopped coriander and serve.

Nutrition

- Calories: 619
- Fat: 41.78g
- Carbohydrate: 41.76g
- Protein: 23.46g

Cranberry Apple Chicken with Cabbage

Servings: 4

Prep Time: 5 mins

Cook Time: 30 mins

Total Time: 35 mins

Ingredients

- 1 small head cabbage, cored and shredded
- 2 pounds boneless, skinless chicken thighs or breasts
- 2 apples, cored and sliced
- 1/2 cup chicken broth (bone broth, if you have it)
- 1 cup fresh or frozen cranberries
- 1 tablespoon apple cider vinegar
- 1 tablespoon maple syrup
- 1 teaspoon cinnamon
- 1 teaspoon ground ginger
- 1/2 teaspoon salt, and more to taste

Instructions

1. Place all ingredients, in the order above, into the Instant Pot. Close lid.
2. Press the Poultry button.
3. Set the time for 20 minutes.
4. Instant Pot will start the cooking process.
5. When cooking has finished, press off button.
6. Allow pressure to release naturally for 10 minutes.
7. Open lid.
8. Serve.

Nutrition

- Calories: 257.1
- Fat: 2.8g
- Carbohydrate: 29.7g
- Protein: 27.9g

Cauli-Rice In The Instant Pot

Servings: 4

Prep Time: 5 mins

Cook Time: 15 mins

Total Time: 20 mins

Ingredients

- 1 medium to large head of cauliflower
- 2 tbs. olive oil
- 1/4 tsp. salt (more to taste)
- 1/2 tsp. dried parsley

Optional seasonings to play with:

- 1/4 tsp. cumin
- 1/4 tsp. turmeric
- 1/4 tsp. paprika
- Fresh cilantro
- Lime wedges (or lime juice)

Instructions

1. Wash cauliflower and trim off the leaves. Usually, this means you'll chop it into a few large pieces.
2. Put all the pieces into the steamer insert in an Instant Pot (or other pressure cooker).
3. Pour one cup of water under the cauliflower and steamer basket.
4. Close and lock the lid. Make sure the valve is closed.
5. Set on manual for one minute. (It will take about 10 minutes to get up to pressure.)
6. After the cook timer beeps, open the valve to quick-release the pressure. (This takes about 2 minutes.)
7. Remove the cauliflower to a plate.
8. Pour out the water in the pot.
9. Return the pot to the cooker and press cancel, then the saute button.
10. Add the oil to the pot, then the cooked cauliflower.
11. Break up with a potato masher.
12. Add desired spices while stirring and heating. Salt and parsley make a pretty basic cauli rice ready for any saucy dish on top.
13. Use the optional spices and serve with fresh cilantro and a squeeze of lime juice for a delicious "cilantro lime" version, or try your own! You can shake a few seasonings in, taste it, and keep trying things.

Nutrition

- Calories: 66
- Fat: 7g
- Carbohydrates: 1.3g
- Protein: .5g

Asian Pork Steaks

Servings: 4-6

Prep time: 5 mins

Cook time: 7 hrs

Total time: 7 hrs 5 mins

Ingredients

- 2-3 lbs bone-in pork steaks
- 1 sweet onion, sliced
- 1/2 cup coconut aminos
- 1/2 cup broth
- 2 tbs honey
- 1 tbs fish sauce
- 4 cloves garlic, finely diced
- 1.5-inch knuckle of ginger, peeled & finely diced

Instructions

1. Place pork steaks and onions in Instant Pot (on slow cooker setting).
2. In a small bowl mix remaining ingredients.
3. Pour mixture over pork.
4. Cover slow cooker and cook on low for 7 hours.
5. Remove pork from slow cooker and place in a large dish.
6. Discard bones (or save them to make broth). Shred the pork with two forks or claws.
7. Drizzle with the remaining liquid.
8. Serve warm over cauliflower rice & steamed vegetables

Nutrition

- Calories: 106.1
- Fat: 5.5g
- Carbohydrate: 2.9g
- Protein: 11.5g

AIP Instant Pot Sweet & Sour Mango Chicken Thighs

Servings: 4

Prep Time: 10 mins

Cook Time: 40 mins

Total Time: 50 mins

Ingredients

- 1 tablespoon cooking fat (I used duck fat)
- 8 chicken thighs, deboned
- 1/2 red onion, chopped
- 1 mango, cut into 1/2 inch chunks
- 4 cloves garlic, chopped
- juice of 1 lime (about 2 tablespoons)
- 1/4 cup + 1 tablespoon coconut aminos, divided
- 1" piece of ginger, chopped finely
- 1/4 cup chopped cilantro
- 2 tablespoons honey
- 1/2 cup chicken broth (bone broth, if you have it)
- 1 teaspoon fish sauce
- 2 tablespoons apple cider vinegar, divided
- 1/2 teaspoon salt
- 1 green onion, sliced (green part only)

Instructions

1- With lid off, press Sauté button on Instant Pot
2- Place cooking fat in the pot.
3- Heat until melted.
4- Place chicken thighs, skin side down, into the pot.
5- Brown for about 3 minutes.
6- Flip thighs over, and brown for about 2 minutes. Depending on the size of your chicken thighs, you may have to do 4 thighs at a time so as not to overcrowd your pot.
7- Remove chicken thighs and set aside.
8- Add onion, mango, and garlic to the pot.
9- Cook until onions are clear and mango has started to brown slightly.
10- Turn off Instant Pot (press Cancel button).
11- Place chicken thighs back into the pot, nestled into mango and onion mixture.
12- Add lime juice, 1/4 cup coconut aminos, ginger, cilantro, honey, chicken broth, fish sauce, and 1 tablespoon apple cider vinegar to the pot.

13- Place lid on Instant Pot. Press the Poultry button, then Pressure button twice, for the high-pressure setting. Timing will set automatically for 15 minutes.
14- Once pressure cooking is done, and Instant Pot goes into Warming mode, turn the pot off.
15- Turn the pressure valve to venting.
16- Be sure all pressure is released from the pot before opening lid.
17- Open lid.
18- Remove chicken thighs from the pot. Set aside.
19- Add 1 tablespoon coconut aminos, 1 tablespoon apple cider vinegar and salt to the pot.
20- Press the Sauté button.
21- Cook sauce until it reduces into a thick sauce; about 10-15 minutes.
22- Turn the pot off.
23- Serve chicken thighs with sauce ladled on top.
24- Add green onion slices for garnish.

Nutrition

- Calories: 183
- Fat: 8g
- Carbohydrate: 13g
- Protein: 13g

AIP Instant Pot Blackberry Balsamic Chicken

Servings: 6

Prep Time: 15 mins

Cook Time: 45 mins

Total Time: 1 hr

Ingredients

- 6 boneless, skinless chicken thighs or breasts
- 16 ounces fresh or frozen blackberries
- 1/4 cup balsamic vinegar
- 1 tablespoon organic molasses
- 1 tablespoon maple syrup
- 2 green onions, sliced
- 2 cloves garlic, chopped
- 1/2 teaspoon salt
- 2 tablespoons arrowroot flour

Instructions

1- Place all ingredients, except arrowroot flour, into Instant Pot.
2- Close lid.
3- Press the "Poultry" button.
4- When done cooking, press "Warm/Cancel".
5- Allow releasing pressure naturally for 10 minutes.
6- Carefully open lid.
7- Remove chicken pieces from Instant Pot, and set aside.
8- Pour blackberry sauce through a mesh strainer into a medium bowl.
9- Stir and mash blackberries to strain out seeds.
10- Pour the strained sauce back into the Instant Pot.
11- Press the "Saute" button, and whisk arrowroot flour into sauce.
12- Cook until sauce thickens; about 10 minutes.
13- Add chicken back into the sauce and warm through for 5 minutes.
14- Press the "Warm/Cancel" button.
15- Serve chicken with sauce ladled on top.

Nutrition

- Calories: 223
- Fat: 7g
- Carbohydrate: 0g
- Protein: 0g

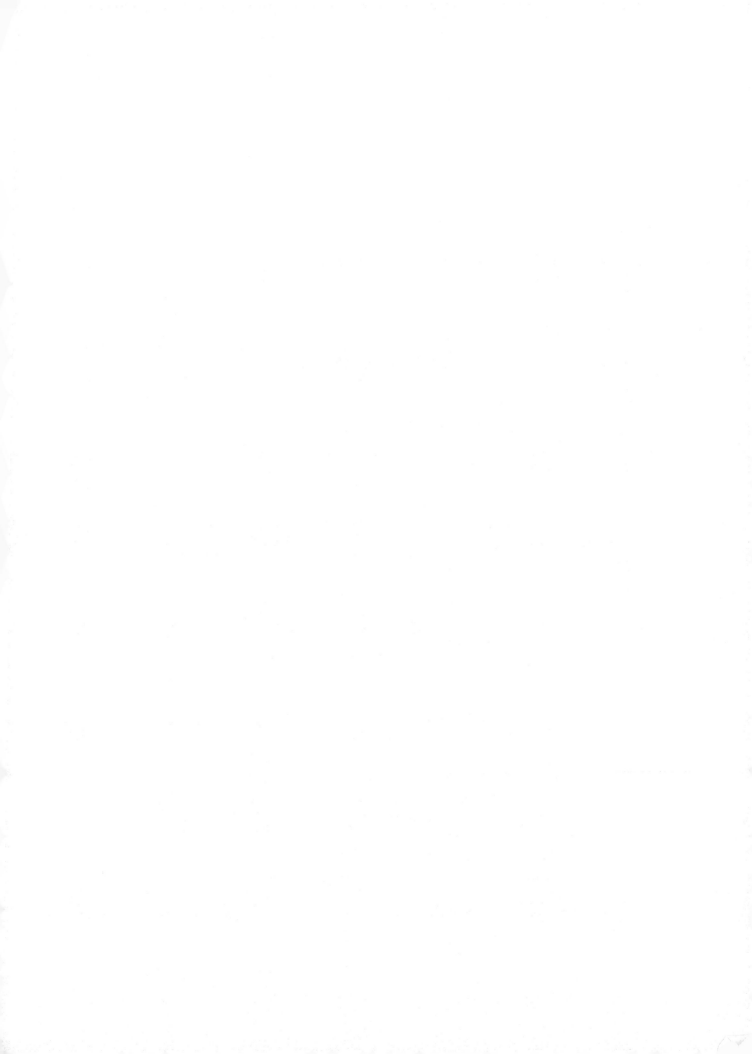

Cranberry Turkey

Servings: 6-8

Prep time: 10 mins

Cook time: 25 mins

Total time: 35 mins

Ingredients

- 2 cups sauerkraut, drained
- ¼ cup raisins
- 3 cloves garlic, peeled, smashed, and roughly chopped
- 3 - 4 lbs (1.5 - 2kg) turkey wings or thighs
- 1.5 cups fresh or frozen cranberries, divided
- 1 small preserved lemon, chopped with seeds removed
- 1 tsp ground cinnamon
- ½ tbsp dried parsley flakes
- 1 tsp dried thyme
- 1 tsp sea salt
- 1 cup apple cider (non-alcoholic hard cider)
- 1 tsp arrowroot flour
- 2 tsp water

Instructions

1. Place the sauerkraut at the bottom of the pot, then scatter the raisins and garlic over evenly
2. Place the turkey parts in the pot
3. Sprinkle 1 cup cranberries and preserved lemon over the turkey parts
4. In a bowl, combine the ground cinnamon, parsley flakes, thyme, sea salt and apple cider and pour into the pot
5. Seal the lid of the pressure cooker (set the valve to 'sealing') and select 'poultry' setting for 25-30 minutes (depending on the size of the turkey parts used)
6. Once the cooking time is over, release the pressure naturally
7. Preheat the oven broiler in the meantime
8. Remove the turkey pieces from the pot and place them in an oven-proof casserole, then broil for around 5 minutes until browned to your liking
9. Set the Instant Pot to 'Saute' setting, then add in another ½ cup of cranberries
10. Prepare the arrowroot flour slurry by combining the arrowroot flour with water
11. Once the sauce begins to simmer, stir in the slurry, then allow the sauce to simmer until thickened
12. Turn off the Instant Pot and serve the cranberry and sauerkraut sauce with the browned turkey

Nutrition

- Calories: 650
- Fat: 18g
- Carbohydrate: 86g
- Protein: 34g

Instant Pot Chicken Taquitos (AIP + Paleo / Whole30)

Servings: 4

Prep Time 10 mins

Cook Time 20 mins

Total Time 30 mins

Ingredients

- 1 lb chicken breasts
- 1/4 cup broth or water
- 1 1/2 tbsp taco seasoning
- 2 tbsp nutritional yeast
- 1/4 tsp sea salt
- 1/2 cup AIP cream cheese

Instructions

1. Place chicken breast, broth or water, taco seasoning, nutritional yeast and sea salt into Instant Pot.
2. Pressure cook on high for 15 minutes.
3. When done, allow to depressurize on its own (takes a few minutes).
4. Remove chicken into glass bowl and shred using two forks.
5. Add 3/4 liquid, discarding the rest.
6. Add cream cheese and mix to combine.
7. Either return to Instant Pot on warm until ready to serve, or enjoy!!

Nutrition

- Calories: 370
- Fat: 17g
- Carbohydrate: 43g
- Protein: 12g

AIP Taco Seasoning

Servings: ½ cup

Prep Time: 5 mins

Cook Time: 0 minutes

Total Time: 5 mins

Ingredients

- 2 1/2 tsp minced dried onion
- 1 tsp cilantro
- 1 tsp turmeric
- 1 tsp garlic
- 3/4 tsp sea salt
- 1/8 tsp cloves
- 1/8 tsp cinnamon

Instructions

1. Place all spices into small bowl.
2. Whisk or stir until fully combined.

Nutrition

- Calories: 20
- Fat: 0g
- Carbohydrate: 4g
- Protein: 0g

Instant Pot Duck Confit

Servings: 4

Prep Time: 24 hours

Cook Time: 2 hours

Total Time: 26 hours

Ingredients

- 1 tablespoon kosher salt
- 4 sprigs fresh thyme
- 4 garlic cloves, smashed
- 2 bay leaves, torn in half
- 1/4 teaspoon black peppercorns, lightly crushed
- 1/4 teaspoon allspice berries, lightly crushed
- 4 duck legs (drumsticks and thighs)

Instructions

1. Line a small-rimmed baking sheet or a plate with paper towels.
2. In a large bowl, stir together the salt, thyme, garlic, bay leaves, peppercorns, and allspice.
3. Add the duck legs and toss, covering the legs evenly with the salt.
4. Place the duck legs in a single layer on the baking sheet and refrigerate, uncovered, for at least 24 hours and up to 3 days.
5. Brush the garlic and thyme sprigs off the duck, reserving them.
6. Using the sauté function, arrange the duck legs, skin-side down, in the pressure cooker, with as much of the flesh touching the bottom of the pot as possible.
7. Sear until the skin turns golden brown and the fat starts to render; around 5 to 10 minutes.
8. Flip the duck legs over and sear on the other side for 5 to 10 minutes.
9. Scatter the reserved garlic and thyme on top of the duck.
10. Cover and cook the duck legs on high pressure for 40 minutes, and then release the pressure manually.
11. Flip the legs over, and cook on high pressure for another 30 minutes.
12. Let the pressure release naturally.
13. Let the duck cool completely, and then store it, covered in its own rendered fat (there will be lots of it in the pot), in the refrigerator.
14. When you are ready to serve, heat the broiler.
15. Scrape fat off duck legs.
16. Transfer the duck to a rimmed baking sheet and broil until the skin is crispy; around 3 to 5 minutes (or you can crisp up the duck in a hot, dry skillet).

Nutrition

- Calories: 318
- Fat: 17.5g
- Carbohydrate: 2.5g
- Protein: 37.6g

Pressure Cooked Cabbage with Minced Pork

Servings: 4-6

Prep Time: 15 minutes

Cook Time: 30 minutes

Total Time: 45 minutes

Ingredients

- 1 tbsp bacon fat/ oil of your choice
- 1 shallot, chopped
- 1 lb lean minced pork
- ½ head medium green cabbage, cut into large bite-sized pieces
- ½ head medium red cabbage, cut into large bite-sized pieces
- 3 cloves garlic, chopped
- ¼ preserved lemon, diced (optional)
- 1 carrot, peeled & sliced diagonally (about ⅓" thick)
- ½ cup bone broth
- Sea salt, to taste
- Coconut aminos or soy-free coconut seasoning, to taste
- 1 sheet toasted seaweed

Instructions

1. Select 'Sauté' setting on your Instant Pot pressure cooker
2. Once the display shows 'Hot', place fat/ oil in the inner pot, add shallots and cook until they start to brown
3. Cooking in batches, add half of the minced pork into the inner pot, allowing it to brown before removing, then cook the other half
4. Add the rest of the ingredients, except for the sea salt and coconut aminos
5. Press 'Keep warm/cancel' setting and cover, sealing the valve
6. Press 'Manual' setting and adjust the cooking time to 3 minutes
7. Once the cooking time is complete, release pressure by quick release method
8. Stir gently to mix and season to taste with sea salt and coconut aminos
9. Garnish with thinly cut strips of seaweed, if desired, and serve

Nutrition

- Calories: 267
- Fat: 12.7g
- Carbohydrate: 15.4g
- Protein: 24.1g

Braised Pork in Soy Sauce (tau yew bak)

Servings: 4

Prep Time: 15 minutes

Cook Time: 40 minutes

Total Time: 55 minutes

Ingredients

- 1 lb. pork belly, cut into small pieces
- 4 cups water
- 1 bulb garlic, lightly pounded with the back of a cleaver
- 1 tablespoon white peppercorn, smashed and cracked
- 5 hard-boiled eggs
- 8 oz. fried tofu/bean curd
- 4 tablespoons soy sauce
- 3 tablespoons sweet soy sauce
- 1-2 tablespoons dark soy sauce
- Salt to taste

Instructions

1. Heat up a pot with 4 cups of water
2. Bring it to boil and then add in the garlic, pork belly, and cracked pepper
3. Bring the pork belly to boil before adding the hard-boiled eggs, fried tofu, soy sauce, sweet soy sauce, and dark soy sauce
4. Lower the heat to medium and braise the pork for 30 minutes or so until the pork bellyis cooked through and become tender. Add salt to taste
5. Continue to simmer on the lowest heat for another 15-20 minutes
6. Dish out and serve hot with steamed white rice

Nutrition

- Calories 611
- Fat 69g
- Carbohydrates 18g
- Protein 26g

Instant Pot Maple Tamarind Ribs

Servings: 4

Prep Time: 10 minutes

Cook Time: 1 hour 5 minutes

Total Time: 1 hour 15 minutes

Ingredients

- 1 rack of baby back pork ribs
- 1 teaspoon fine sea salt
- 1 teaspoon garlic powder
- 1 teaspoon dried thyme
- 1/4 cup liquid (broth or water)
- 2 tablespoons maple syrup
- 1 tablespoon tamarind paste

Instructions

1. Mix together the salt, garlic and thyme and rub on both sides of the rack of ribs until well seasoned.
2. Slice the rack of ribs into three equal-sized portions and lay them in the bottom of the Instant Pot.
3. Pour the liquid around (not on top of) the ribs.
4. Set the Instant Pot to cook on the "Manual" setting for 50 minutes.
5. Let pressure release naturally when timer goes off.
6. Whisk together the maple and tamarind until combined and heat your oven broiler to 425 degrees. Arrange the top oven rack 6 to 8 inches away from the broiler element.
7. Place the cooked ribs on a rimmed baking sheet meaty side up and baste with half of the maple-tamarind sauce.
8. Broil for 5 to 7 minutes until bubbling and caramelized, remove from oven, and baste with additional maple-tamarind sauce.
9. Broil for another 3 to 5 minutes until caramelized.
10. Season with additional sea salt and serve immediately.

Nutrition

- Calories: 301
- Fat: 19g
- Carbohydrate: 8g
- Protein: 22g

Pressure Cooker Sweet & Tangy Pulled Pork

Servings: 4

Prep Time: 10 minutes

Cook Time: 40 minutes

Total Time: 50 minutes

Ingredients

- 2 lbs boneless pork roast
- 1 tablespoon fat of choice
- 12 oz fresh or frozen cranberries
- 10 oz bone broth of choice
- 2 tablespoons chopped fresh herbs of choice
- 2 tablespoons apple cider vinegar
- 1 tablespoon honey
- 1/4 tsp ground cinnamon
- 1/8 teaspoon ground cloves

Instructions

1. Set your Instant Pot to the sauté function.
2. Pour fat of choice into the bottom of the pot and spread it around with a spatula.
3. Salt pork generously on all sides and place in hot oil.
4. Sear on each side, uncovered, for 2 minutes until lightly browned.
5. Set the Instant Pot to the Manual pressure cooker setting for 70 minutes.
6. Add cranberries and broth to the bottom of pot, being sure not to "wash away" the salt off the pork. Sprinkle chopped herbs, apple cider vinegar and honey on top and close the lid.
7. Cook undisturbed for full 70 minutes.
8. Release the pressure using the release valve, remove the pork to a cutting board and use two forks to shred the pork.
9. Place back in the Instant Pot, sprinkle with a pinch more sea salt, and set the manual option for another 10 minutes.
10. This allows the shredded pork to absorb the broth, increasing its moisture and flavor.
11. Remove pork and cranberries from the liquid and place in a large serving dish.
12. Toss with the cinnamon, garlic, and cloves and serve warm.

Nutrition

- Calories: 400
- Fat: 8g
- Carbohydrate: 50g
- Protein: 27g

4-Ingredient Multi-Purpose Instant Pot Shredded Beef

Servings: 6

Prep Time: 2 mins

Cook Time: 1 hr

Total Time: 1 hr 2 mins

Ingredients

- 3-4 lb of beef rump roast or chuck roast
- 1 tsp sea salt
- 2 tbsp coconut oil
- 2 1/2 cups of bone broth or beef broth

Instructions

1. Cut the roast into 4 even pieces and season all sides with salt.
2. Set Instant Pot to the Sauté setting and heat coconut oil in the pot for 10 minutes.
3. Add the roast pieces and brown on all sides, about 10 minutes.
4. Press Cancel, and add the broth over the beef.
5. Close the lid and make sure the pressure-release valve is closed.
6. Cook at high pressure on Manual for 50 minutes.
7. Once the Instant Pot beeps to signal that it's done, let it sit for 10-15 minutes to allow the pressure to release naturally until the lid opens.
8. Transfer the roast to a cutting board, and shred the meat with 2 forks.
9. Return to the Instant Pot and keep warm until ready to use.
10. You can eat the shredded beef on its own with various sides, or use it in other dishes like tacos, burrito bowls, stir-frys, sandwiches, and more.

Nutrition

- Calories: 271.4
- Fat: 7.8g
- Carbohydrate: 10.1g
- Protein: 36.1g

Instant Pot Beef Bourgignon

Servings: 4

Prep time: 20 mins

Cook time: 40 mins

Total time: 1 hr

Ingredients

- 1 pound of stewing beef or flank steak, cubed
- ½ pound of bacon
- 5 medium carrots, roughly chopped
- 1 large red onion, roughly chopped
- 2 cloves garlic
- 2 teaspoons sea salt
- 2 teaspoons dried thyme
- 2 teaspoons dried parsley
- 2 teaspoons ground black pepper (omit if on AIP elimination)
- 1 cup red wine
- ½ cup beef bone broth
- 1 tablespoon avocado oil or olive oil
- 2 large sweet potatoes/kumara
- 1 tablespoon maple syrup

Instructions

1. Switch Instant Pot to 'browning' setting
2. Add oil
3. Pat beef dry and season. Sauté in batches to give them room in the Instant Pot to brown
4. Set aside
5. Slice bacon into thin strips and brown with onions
6. Add browned beef and then add all remaining ingredients
7. Switch Instant Pot to 'high pressure' setting and set to 40 minutes
8. Spoon into bowls and enjoy!

Nutrition

- Calories: 442.4
- Fat: 17.3g
- Carbohydrate: 16.1g
- Protein: 39.8g

Instant Pot Mongolian Beef

Servings: 6

Prep time: 10 mins

Cook time: 10 mins

Total time: 20 mins

Ingredients

- 1.5 pounds flank steak
- 3/4 cup brown sugar
- 3/4 cup soy sauce
- 2 cloves garlic
- 3/4 cup beef broth
- 2 tbs corn starch
- 2 tbs sesame oil
- 1 cup shredded carrots

Instructions

1. Place pot on Saute.
2. Add oil, steak, and garlic.
3. Pour in carrots, soy sauce, brown sugar, and broth.
4. Cook on Manual High pressure 10 minutes
5. Quick Release.
6. Place pot back on Saute, and bring to a boil
7. Whisk in cornstarch.
8. Continue on Sauté for about 2-3 minutes until sauce thickens

Nutrition

- Calories: 383
- Total fat: 14g
- Carbohydrates: 28g
- Protein: 35g

Instant Pot Beef Brisket

Servings: 4

Prep time: 45mins

Cook time: 55 mins

Total time: 1hr 40m

Ingredients

- 1 onion
- 2 cloves garlic
- 1 tbsp. bacon fat, or fat of choice
- 1 tsp. coarse sea salt, or to taste
- 1 tsp. garlic powder
- 1 tsp. onion powder
- 1/2 tsp. dried oregano
- 1/2 tsp. dried thyme
- 1/4 c beef stock, or chicken stock
- 1 tbsp. sucanat
- 2 lb beef brisket

Instructions

1. Peel and slice the onion.
2. Peel and halve the garlic.
3. Turn the pressure cooker to Sauté.
4. Sauté onion and garlic in fat until translucent.
5. Stir in spices and seasoning
6. Cook for 2 minutes. Remove and set aside.
7. In the bottom of your pressure cooker, loosely combine the stock and sucanat.
8. Place brisket in the pressure cooker and spread onion mixture over the top.
9. Cover with the lid and cook on high pressure for 50 minutes.
10. Once cooking is complete, you can quick release pressure or natural release.
11. When the brisket is cooked but still hot, use a spoon to scrape off any large fat deposits adhered to the top and bottom of the brisket.
12. Transfer the brisket and all of its sauce to a baking dish.
13. Chill entire dish in the fridge for several hours and up to one day; this resting time will significantly enhance the flavor and texture of the meat.
14. Remove the dish from the fridge and remove as much solidified fat as you'd.
15. Move the meat to a cutting board and slice against the grain into half-inch slices.
16. Use an immersion blender (or standing blender) to puree the sauce until smooth.

17. Slide the sliced meat back and sauce back into the pressure cooker on high for 3 minutes to warm. Use manual or natural release.
18. Serve with a simple, fresh salad.

Nutrition

- Calories: 403
- Protein: 47g
- Carbs: 7g
- Fats: 16g

Tender Herb Crusted Pot Roast (Instant Pot, AIP/Paleo)

Servings: 4-5

Prep Time: 20 minutes

Cook Time: 1 hour 10 minutes

Total Time: 1 hour 30 minutes

Ingredients

- 2 tbs cooking fat (coconut oil works great)
- 1-1.5 lb chuck eye or sirloin tip roast
- 1 cup water
- 5 tsp granulated garlic
- 1 tsp dried oregano
- 1 tsp Himalayan pink salt
- 1 tsp dried rosemary
- ½ tsp dried basil
- ¼ tsp dried thyme
- 2 tsp olive oil

Instructions

1. Press Sauté on your Instant Pot and wait for it to heat up.
2. Place the cooking oil in the liner and lightly brown all sides of your roast,
3. Once browned, press "Off".
4. Pour in 1 cup of water, making sure the top of the meat is not submerged (you may need to pour in a little less).You may need to pour in a little less.
5. Blend your seasonings and olive oil in a small bowl to form a paste
6. Once blended, cover the top of the meat with the paste.
7. Allow some bits to fall into the water – this will infuse the flavor into the meat as it cooks.
8. Press the "Meat/Stew" option and "Adjust".
9. Adjust the time to 45 minutes.
10. Allow to naturally release, which takes about 30 minutes.
11. Slice on the thin side and enjoy!

Nutrition

- Calories: 209
- Fat: 10.3g
- Carbohydrate: 0g
- Protein: 26.8g

Chapter 10:
Seafood Recipes

Instant Pot Steamed Crab Legs

Servings: 4

Prep Time: 1 minute

Cook Time: 2 minutes

Total Time: 3 minutes

Ingredients

- 3 clusters fresh crab legs
- 1 cup water

Instructions

1. Insert steaming rack into your Instant Pot.
2. Pour 1 cup of water.
3. Add fresh or thawed crab legs (if using frozen) to the pot.
4. Place the lid on the Instant Pot and seal the vent.
5. Press the manual button and set the time to 2 minutes.
6. Once the Instant Pot beeps, quick release the pressure.
7. Use tongs to remove the crab legs.

Nutrition

- Calories: 300
- Fat: 4g
- Carbohydrate: 1g
- Protein: 61g

Easy Coconut Red Curry Shrimp

Servings: 6

Prep time: 5 mins

Cook time: 25 mins

Total time: 30 mins

Ingredients

For the Marinade:

- 1/4 cup coconut milk canned
- 1 tsp cumin
- 1 tsp paprika
- 2 tsp curry spice
- 3 tbsp fresh lime juice
- 1/2 tsp sea salt
- 1 tsp freshly grated ginger
- 1 clove garlic minced
- 2 lbs large shrimp peeled and deveined

For the Sauce:

- 2 tbsp coconut oil or olive oil
- 1 small white onion, diced
- 2 tsp freshly grated ginger
- 2 cloves garlic, minced
- 1 28 oz can of diced tomatoes
- 3 tbsp red Thai curry paste
- 1 14 oz coconut milk
- 1 tsp sea salt
- 1/3 cup freshly chopped cilantro for garnish - optional

Instructions

1. Begin by making your marinade.
2. Place coconut milk, spices, lime juice, sea salt, ginger, and garlic in a large bowl.
3. Whisk together, then add shrimp.
4. Toss to coat and let sit while you prepare the sauce.
5. Select the Sauté function on your Instant Pot.
6. Once hot, add oil to coat the bottom of the pan.
7. Now add onion, ginger, and garlic. Let sauté for a few minutes, then select cancel.
8. Now add tomatoes, curry paste, coconut milk, and salt.

9. Place lid on the IP and secure it.
10. Make sure the valve is sealed. Select the Manual function, and cook on high pressure for 7 minutes.
11. Once the sauce is complete, use the quick-release on your IP.
12. Remove the lid once all the steam has been released, then select cancel.
13. Now select Sauté function, and add in shrimp plus the juices from the marinade.
14. Simmer until the shrimp is cooked through and no longer pink; about 2-5 minutes.
15. Serve with optional cilantro, salt to taste, and over rice or cauliflower rice.

Nutrition

- Calories: 197.5
- Fat: 6.1g
- Carbohydrate: 9.2g
- Protein: 25.6g

Instant Pot Lemon Garlic Salmon (From Frozen!)

Servings: 3-4

Prep Time: 3 mins

Cook Time: 17 mins

Total Time: 20 mins

Ingredients:

- 1 1/2 pounds frozen salmon filets
- 1/4 cup lemon juice
- 3/4 cup water
- A few springs of fresh dill, basil, parsley or a mix
- 1/4 teaspoon garlic powder or to taste (or 2 cloves garlic, minced)
- 1/4 teaspoon sea salt or to taste
- 1/8 teaspoon black pepper
- 1 lemon, sliced thinly
- 1 tablespoon avocado oil or melted coconut oil

Instructions

1. Pour water and lemon juice into your Instant Pot.
2. Add fresh herbs to the water/lemon juice mixture and place steamer rack in Instant Pot.
3. Drizzle salmon with oil and season with salt and pepper.
4. Sprinkle garlic powder over the salmon and place it on the salmon in a single layer on the steamer rack in the Instant Pot.
5. Layer lemon slices on top of the salmon.
6. Place the lid on the Instant Pot, lock in place and turn the valve to sealing. Use the Manual setting to cook on high pressure for 7 minutes.
7. It will take your Instant Pot about 10 minutes to get up to pressure.
8. Once the time is up, switch the valve to venting to quickly release the pressure
9. Enjoy warm over a salad, with roasted veggies or any other way that you can dream up!

Nutrition

- Calories: 201.9
- Fat: 6.7g
- Carbohydrate: 1.8g
- Protein: 31.8g

Seafood Chowder [AIP - Allergy Free - No Shellfish]

Servings: 4

Prep Time: 5 minutes

Cook Time: 25 minutes

Total Time: 30 minutes

Ingredients

- 3 tablespoons extra virgin olive oil
- 3 carrots (about 8 ounces), peeled and diced
- 3 celery ribs (about 5 ounces), finely chopped
- 1 small fennel bulb (about 8 ounces), finely chopped
- 1 small white sweet potato (about 8 ounces), peeled and diced
- 1 1/2 tablespoons minced fresh thyme, plus extra for garnish
- 1 bay leaf
- 1-quart bone broth
- 1/3 pound skinless cod fillet (no thicker than 1 inch)
- 1/3 pound skinless salmon fillet (no thicker than 1 inch)
- 1/2 cup full-fat coconut milk
- Fine sea salt, to taste

Instructions

1. Heat the olive oil in a stockpot over medium heat.
2. Add the carrots, celery, fennel, sweet potato, thyme, and bay leaf.
3. Sauté, stirring frequently, for about 10 minutes, until crisp-tender. (Don't let the vegetables brown or stick to the bottom of the pot.
4. If needed, reduce the heat or add an extra drizzle of olive oil.)
5. Add the bone broth to the pot and bring to a boil over high heat.
6. Reduce the heat to medium.
7. Add the cod and salmon.
8. Cook for 8 to 10 minutes, until the vegetables are tender and the fish is cooked through.
9. Discard the bay leaf and transfer the fish to a plate with a slotted spatula.
10. Break the fish into smaller pieces, discarding any stray fish bones you find.
11. Return the fish to the pot.
12. Stir in the coconut milk and season with sea salt to taste.
13. Garnish with minced fresh thyme right before serving piping hot.

Nutrition

- Calories: 510
- Fat: 38g

- Carbohydrate: 31g
- Protein: 20g

Shrimp Etouffee

Servings: 4

Prep Time: 1 hour 30 minutes

Cook Time: 30 minutes

Total Time: 2 hours

Ingredients

- 3 tbsp lard
- 1 small sweet onion, diced
- 1 stalk celery, diced
- 1/2 bell pepper, diced (AIP: sub 1 more stalk celery or 1 small carrot)
- 1/4 cup cassava flour
- 2 large cloves garlic, pressed
- 1 tbsp Cajun seasoning (AIP: sub 1/2 tsp garlic powder, 1/2 tsp onion powder, 1/4 tsp Italian seasoning, 1 tsp ginger powder, 1 tsp horseradish powder, and 1/4 tsp Himalayan salt)
- 1 tbsp dried parsley
- 1/2 tsp Himalayan salt
- 1 to 2 tsp Frank's Red Hot (AIP: sub 1 to 2 tsp lemon juice)
- 3 cups bone broth fish, chicken or pork
- 1 bay leaf
- 1 lb medium shrimp peeled, deveined, tails removed and strained very well (you can also use crawfish, cubed skinless fish or scallops)
- lemon wedges

Instructions

1. Press Sauté. When the display reads Hot, add the lard, onion, celery and bell pepper. Stir well.
2. Cook, stirring occasionally, for 7 minutes or until browned and slightly caramelized.
3. Press Cancel, then vigorously stir in cassava flour until mixture binds together. Stir in garlic, Cajun seasoning, parsley, salt, and hot sauce.
4. Press Sauté. Press Adjust until Lessis illuminated.
5. Drizzle in 1 cup of the bone broth, stirring continuously to prevent lumps. When the mixture is smooth, slowly add the remaining 2 cups broth while stirring, then add the bay leaf.
6. Bring to a simmer, stirring and scraping the bottom every couple of minutes to prevent sticking. Cook this way for 10 to 15 minutes, or until sauce is thickened and reduced to 2/3.
7. Stir in shrimp. Cook for 2 minutes, stirring continuously. Press Cancel.
8. (Shrimp will continue to cook slightly in the hot gravy, so it is best to stop the heat underneath just before they look completely done.)
9. Serve in bowls with lemon wedges and a splash of hot sauce.

Nutrition

- Calories: 185.2
- Fat: 12.4g
- Carbs: 5.8g
- Protein: 13.2g

Chapter 11: Dessert Recipes

Mini Crustless Pumpkin Pies / Fresh Pumpkin Pie Filling

Serves: 1-8

Prep time: 5 mins

Cook time: 15 mins

Total time: 20 mins

Ingredients

- 2 lbs (1k) butternut squash, peeled and diced (or one 2-3lb sugar pumpkin, seeded and cut into manageable chunks - see special notes)
- 1 cup (250ml) whole milk (or fresh cream, or coconut milk)
- ¾ cup maple (185ml) 100% pure maple syrup
- 2 large eggs
- 1 teaspoon powdered cinnamon
- ½ teaspoon powdered ginger (or 1" piece fresh ginger, peeled & very finely chopped)
- ¼ teaspoon powdered cloves
- 1 tablespoon organic corn starch
- 2 pinches sea salt

Garnish:

- sweetened whipped cream
- chopped pecans

Instructions

1. Prepare the pressure cooker by adding 1 cup (250ml) water, or your pressure cooker's minimum liquid requirement, and add the squash cubes to the steamer basket and lower into the pressure cooker.
2. Close the lid and set the valve to the pressure cooking position.
3. Electric pressure cookers: Cook for 4 minutes at high pressure (9 minutes for wedges).
4. Stovetop pressure cookers: Lock the lid, and cook for 3 minutes at high pressure (7 minutes for wedges).
5. In the meantime, in a 4-cup measuring cup (a 1L pitcher), or medium mixing bowl, measure out the milk, maple syrup, and then add the eggs, cinnamon, ginger, salt, and cornstarch. Beat, using a fork or an immersion blender, until the ingredients are well combined.
6. When the pressure cooking time is up, open the cooker by releasing the pressure through the valve.
7. Tumble the cooked butternut squash in a fine-mesh strainer (or peel the cooked pumpkin and then strain) and once cooled (about 10 minutes) press on the squash pulp to release some liquid (save this liquid to use in place of stock in other recipes).

8. Measure the strained pumpkin pulp by jamming it into a 2-cup measure (or weighing out 550g) - measure out and freeze or refrigerate the rest for future pumpkin pies or to plop into a pasta sauce or soup.
9. Plop the pulp into the measuring cup with the egg mixture and blend well.
   To make cute crust-less pies in the pressure cooker:
10. Add 1 cup (250ml) water, or your pressure cooker's minimum liquid requirement, to the pressure cooker and steamer basket or trivet and set aside.
11. Pour the mixture into heat-proof ramekins and lower into the pressure cooker uncovered - put the second layer on top of the first by balancing on the edges of the ramekins below.
12. Close the lid and set the valve to the pressure cooking position.
13. Electric pressure cookers: Cook for 10 minutes at high pressure.
14. Stovetop pressure cookers: Lock the lid, and cook for 8 minutes at high pressure.
15. When time is up, open the pressure cooker with the 10-Minute Natural release method - move the cooker off the burner and wait for the pressure to come down on its own (about 10 minutes). For electric pressure cookers, when cooking time is up count 10 minutes of natural open time. Then, release the rest of the pressure slowly using the valve.
16. Lift the ramekins out of the pressure cooker using tongs and let stand 5 minutes before serving or let cool completely; cover tightly and refrigerate for up to two days.
17. To fill a pre-cooked pie crust and bake:
18. Preheat oven to 350°F/180°C
19. Pour filling into a 9-inch baked pie crust and cover the edges only with a ring of foil. Bake on the center rack until the center of the pie is just set (a clean toothpick comes out of the center), which will take 45 to 50 minutes.
20. Serve with whipped cream and chopped pecans sprinkled on top.

Nutrition

- Calories: 143.9
- Fat: 2.3g
- Carbohydrate: 2.1g
- Protein: 3.3g

Instant Pot Coconut Yogurt (AIP)

Servings: 1.5 cups (350 ml)

Prep Time: 10 mins

Cook Time: 9 hrs

Total Time: 9 hours 10 minutes

Ingredients

- 3 14-oz cans of coconut milk, refrigerated
- 4 capsules of probiotics
- 2 tablespoons (14 g) gelatin (for thickening)
- 1 tablespoon (15 ml) maple syrup or honey (to enable the yogurt to be made)

Instructions

1. Use a spoon to remove the solid cream on top of the cans of coconut milk.
2. Place this into the instant pot bowl.
3. Close the lid, make sure the vent is closed, press the yogurt button, press Adjust until it shows Boil.
4. When the instant pot is done, it'll beep.
5. Remove the bowl from the instant pot and let cool.
6. Use a candy or meat thermometer to see when the mixture reaches around 100 F (38 C).
7. Open up the capsules of probiotics and slowly whisk them into the coconut cream.
8. Place the bowl back into the instant pot, close the lid, press Yogurt and press (+) to set the time to 8 hours.
9. Add the yogurt to a blender and slowly add the gelatin while blending.
10. Refrigerate for a few hours to cool and thicken.

Nutrition

- Calories: 110
- Fat: 7g
- Carbohydrate: 10g
- Protein: <1g

Instant Pot Paleo Chocolate Chip Banana Bread

Servings: 1-2

Prep Time: 15 mins

Cook Time: 55 mins

Total Time: 1 hr 10 mins

Ingredients

- 1/2 cup avocado oil or grass-fed butter, room temperature
- 1/2 cup maple syrup or light-colored honey
- 3 very ripe small organic bananas, quartered
- 2 pastured or organic eggs, room temperature
- 1 teaspoon vanilla extract
- 1 1/4 cup Otto's cassava flour
- 1/4 cup hydrolyzed grass-fed collagen - optional
- 1 teaspoon baking soda
- 1/2 teaspoon Celtic sea salt
- 1/2 cup stevia-sweetened chocolate chips, allergy-friendly chocolate chips or chopped fair trade organic chocolate

Instructions

1. Grease a 1 1/2 quart covered casserole dish and set aside.
2. In a blender, add all ingredients (except for the chocolate chips) in the order listed, cover and blend on low speed for about 20-30 seconds or until fully combined
3. Pour the batter into the greased casserole dish and cover with the glass lid.
4. Add 1 cup of water into your Instant Pot and place the Instant Pot trivet inside the pot.
5. Carefully set the covered casserole dish inside the Instant Pot on top of the trivet.
6. Put the Instant Pot lid on and secure it in the locked position.
7. When the Instant Pot is done cooking, it will beep to let you know. Allow the Instant Pot to naturally pressure release for 20 minutes.
8. Using an oven mitt, turn the vent to "venting" to manually release any leftover pressure
9. Carefully remove the lid.
10. Using an oven mitt, carefully remove the casserole dish and place it on a cooling rack. Carefully remove the lid (remember it's hot too!)
11. Allow cooling at room temperature for at least 45 minutes.
12. Once the banana bread has thoroughly cooled, cut into thick slices.
13. Enjoy!

Nutrition

- Calories: 398

- Fat: 20g
- Carbohydrates: 57g
- Protein: 15g

Tatin-Style Apple and Lavender Upside-Down Cake

Servings: 6

Prep time: 10 mins

Cook time: 25 mins

Total time: 35 mins

Ingredients

- 2 cups of water
- 4 small Gala apples (about 1⅓ pounds), peeled and cut into ¼-inch slices
- 2 tablespoons lemon juice
- ½ teaspoon dried lavender flowers
- ½ cup tiger nut flour
- ⅓ cup cassava flour
- 2 tablespoons coconut flour
- ½ teaspoon baking powder (or ⅛ teaspoon baking soda + ¼ teaspoon cream of tartar)
- Pinch fine sea salt
- ⅓ cup palm shortening, melted
- 3 tablespoons maple syrup
- 1 teaspoon vanilla extract
- 1 tablespoon gelatin powder

Instructions

1. Add water to the Instant Pot and insert the steaming basket in the pot.
2. Line the bottom of the cake pan with parchment paper.
3. In a dish, mix apples, lemon juice, and lavender together.
4. Spread apples evenly in the bottom of the cake pan.
5. In a large bowl, combine tiger nut flour, cassava flour, coconut flour, baking powder, salt.
6. In a separate bowl, mix together palm shortening, maple syrup, and vanilla extract. Stir well.
7. Sprinkle gelatin powder over palm shortening mixture and whisk vigorously until well blended.
8. Pour liquid mixture over dry ingredients and mix well with a spatula to form a ball of dough.
9. Transfer dough to a piece of parchment paper and flatten with your finger to form a circle no bigger than the cake pan.
10. Cover apples with dough and discard the parchment paper.
11. Cover the cake pan with a piece of aluminum foil, tucking it in all around the rim to create a tight seal.
12. Place the cake pan in the steaming basket. Close and lock the lid. Press "Manual" and cook on high pressure for 25 minutes.
13. When time is up, press cancel and let the pressure release naturally before opening the lid.
14. You can serve this apple tea cake hot or cold.

15. To serve, turn the cake pan upside down and unmold on a serving platter. Eat as is or with a scoop of vanilla ice cream.

Nutrition

- Calories: 236.5
- Fat: 7.7g
- Carbohydrate: 40.3g
- Protein: 4.2g

CONCLUSION

The autoimmune protocol diet can be a strict protocol to follow, but the rewards can pay off big time.

My goal is to support you in making healthy changes so that you can change your life. Never forget; you are strong enough to make the difficult changes required to transform your health.

The introductory AIP diet is highly restrictive, and for some people with autoimmunity, it doesn't need to be followed forever. That's why it's so important to take steps to personalize your AIP diet. Leave a review on Amazon and let us know your experience.

Made in the USA
Monee, IL
06 April 2023

31436230R00103